ARGUE ABORTION

AND OTHER REPRODUCTIVE ISSUES

Like a Doc'

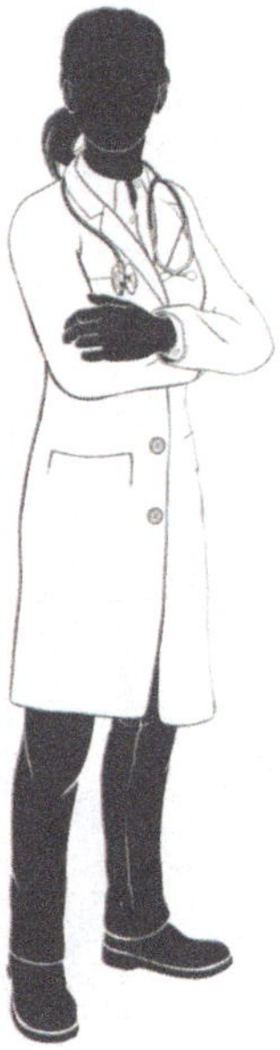

WRITTEN BY
NICOLE RYAN

Table of Contents

Introduction:

When I was a second year medical student, Roe v. Wade was still in existence and I was planning on going into family medicine one day. My dream was to finish med school, get myself through residency, and eventually open a practice with flexible hours for busy families. I wanted to be able to provide the type of care that extended from babies with ear infections, to children who aren't meeting developmental milestones, to women who have questions about rising syphilis rates. I was minding my own business, finishing up reproduction and endocrinology exams when American news exploded with abortion debates. As desperation kicked in and the overturn of Roe v. Wade approached, both sides of the argument started grasping at straws. Democrats and Republicans alike started saying crazy sh** about women's bodies. There's no other way to put it; things got weird. Female politicians were claiming rape is less likely to cause pregnancy than consentual sex,[1] a judge had to do an embryology lesson in her courtroom, someone suggested women should swallow a camera to

[1]Paybarah, A. (2022, June 28). *G.O.P. house candidate falsely suggests pregnancy from rape is unlikely.* The New York Times. https://www.nytimes.com/2022/06/27/us/politics/yesli-vega-rape-pregnant.html

inspect their pregnancies. And those are just examples from the American government. My friends' Facebook feeds were even more bizarre.

For the first time in my life, I was armed with a deeper academic understanding of a topic than the general public. As a former college drop-out, how did this happen?

I always liked science, but it was an easier path for me to build a career in Communications when I was younger so that's the way I went. Occasionally I tried going to college, but I always found the real world more exciting (and a lot more profitable) than the school-world. Over time I did a bit of everything including content writing, training, marketing, and starting a business. I made my connections and made my money (selling a healthcare education company will do that), but I still had more than half of my working life in front of me. I finally finished that partially completed undergrad degree and entered medical school as the Coronavirus pandemic neared an end. At the time, I thought working in medicine would be a good way to feel useful over the next few decades. Instead, I discovered I loved scientific academia. I always thought I knew a fair amount about certain topics because I'd worked in healthcare adjacent fields and had my EMT license. Obviously I wasn't a doctor, but I knew something.

Turns out, that's not really how that works. I quickly realized that so much of medicine and pharmacology is locked behind ivory gates with almost no access to non-medical professionals. I'd always had to rely on popular science websites and magazines when writing an article or researching a topic, but all of a sudden I had logins to research databases and could read original papers. It turns out the original research wasn't always summarized accurately in the popular articles I'd been reading. I also discovered pretty quickly that all the biochemistry and microanatomy we learn in the pre-clinical years of medical school is useful. Actually useful. You can't really understand why birth control works if you don't know at least a little bit about ligand-receptor interactions and hormone pathways. Unfortunately, most writers who deal with science related topics don't delve into these details since it's easier to write in general terms.

Nowadays I find it frustrating that so many of my friends, despite being extremely well read, just don't have the same access to information as I do. Because of that, someone arguing about abortion might say, "but we should give the fetus a chance to live!" not realizing that in the case of a complete molar pregnancy, there is no fetus, only a clump of cells growing out of control (if that sentence doesn't make sense to you, don't worry, it will after you read this book). My point being that we don't give the average person enough information. In fact, when you look up what type of pregnancies are "non-viable" on Google, you'll find thousands of articles, but almost all of them give such a broad overview of complications that if you were to form an opinion based on that information alone, a person with even limited access to proper medical knowledge/data would tear your argument apart in a few seconds.

I, personally, think that's unfair. It should be the duty of medical professionals to share accurate, detailed information about the processes that occur in our bodies when friends, family and/or patients show an interest. That educational process doesn't need to be boring. It can have pictures, questions, even jokes. At the end of the day, medicine is not extremely complicated, it's just detailed[2] and a good instructor should be able to teach details to anyone if they go slow enough.

That's why I wrote this book. I want everyone to have access to the details. Especially people who regularly argue about reproductive rights and regulation.

My dream is to have this book in every politician's office as they prepare for abortion debates on the Senate or Congress floor. On the flip side,

[2] *So* detailed. Seriously, all medical students do for the first two years of school is memorize millions of details about everything ever discovered related to medicine.

when someone confidently proclaims a baby floats around in a uterus, completely unattached to the mother (a thing that actually happened), this book could be condescendingly gifted with a note that says, "it looks like you need to go back and study your biology!"

In fact, if you're a Senator or Congressman, please, for my own enjoyment, carry this book around in your pocket until someone opposed to you says something silly about female anatomy. Then gently drop it on the counter and be proud of yourself for top tier passive aggressive point-making.

When a future bill threatens to reinstate Roe v. Wade laws, I want to step onto the NYC subway and see hordes of normal people holding this book in their laps as they stare off into space considering how they feel about one of the many "questions to ponder" you'll find in text boxes throughout the following pages. My goal isn't to tell anyone what conclusion to draw, but to help debaters draw medically accurate conclusions in the first place.

I truly believe that on both sides of every debate there are points that need to be made and arguments that need to be heard, but those arguments get lost if they're entirely inaccurate. The person arguing also tends to become a meme if what they said was bad enough, and that's something we'd all like to avoid.

Overall, I believe it's every citizen's duty to elevate the discussion when it comes to policy change or medical regulation. Challenge your friends to read an academic article or original research paper. If you don't work in academia, services like DeepDyve can help you access peer reviewed journals so you can get past the gatekeeping of medical knowledge. Double check facts using original data as your standard. Explain that randomized control trials and meta analyses are better sources than singular case reports and for goodness sake, repeat this mantra: Replication equals reliability. If anyone gives you a small one-off study that's never been replicated as concrete evidence for a point, acknowledge the shortcomings of that source.

So in the spirit of elevating arguments, I suggest a fun challenge. For everyone out there living your best life on social media, try out the hashtags #knowyouranatomy and #ThatsNotHowThatWorks. Go forth and use these liberally whenever you see someone claim that women can just pause menstruation, or state that there's no way to become pregnant if someone uses birth control. When another person claims that Plan B kills a fetus, be ready with #ThatsNotHowThatWorks because, guess what? It's not. And we all have a responsibility to clarify things.

Peeling back the curtain on publishing and reviews
Just like I wrote this book to make medical information more accessible, I'm adding this small blob of text to do the same for writing and publishing.

Is it annoying that writers are always asking for reviews and 5 star ratings? Yes.
Is it easier to read a book and move on without going back to the Amazon page and finding the "write a review" button? Yes. 100 times yes.

However, with the rise of the self-published writer and now, AI generated content, it's nearly impossible to get attention for a new book. How does someone differentiate between an AI created how-to book, a poorly edited self help guide, and a professionally edited book written by an expert in their field? Reviews. Reviews and ratings. The more ratings, reviews, and reads a book has, the more likely websites like Amazon are to include that book in suggested listings. Additionally, many blogs and book review platforms only include books that have a specified number of reviews and a minimum rating level (for example,

20+ reviews with a 4.5+ rating). However, getting a book mentioned on blogs and review platforms is one of the main ways to get those reviews. It's a classic Catch-22 situation. Add in the fact that literary agents now ask for sales numbers and ratings for previously written books, and those 4 and 5 star acknowledgements become even more important. After all, being a self published writer with huge sales and good reviews is a great way to attract literary agents for future releases. And you can't get in front of a traditional publisher without an agent.

So please, review, share, rate this book or any other book you're reading on Amazon/Google/wherever. If you're an active GoodReads user, do the same. If you hate a book, that's OK, be honest. But maybe attach that honesty to a 3 star rating because at least there aren't any typos (and if there are, let me know so I can tell my editor).

And if you're on Twitter, Facebook, TikTok, or Instagram, share what you're reading! Buying an independently published book is a great way to support new authors, and sharing the love on social platforms is a great way to amplify that support. Even if you aren't compelled to do so for this book, keep in mind how much power you have as a reader to make or break a new writer and use that power for good!

Go forth and rate, review, share, support.

Chapter 1
Female Reproductive System

For those of you who came into this world equipped with a uterus, it may be tempting to skip this chapter. However, I've heard multiple female politicians imply that the reproductive tract can physically close itself off to unwanted intruders, so let's all do a quick review for accuracy.

What is the reproductive system?
The female reproductive system is self-contained with the main point of entry safely nestled between a person's legs. It's comprised of four main parts: the vagina, uterus/cervix, fallopian tubes, and ovaries. I like to imagine it as a meaty version of a Texas Longhorn silhouette (no relation to any specific college or university). The horns are the fallopian tubes and the face is the uterus. Now imagine the longhorn cow is drinking

through a straw – that's the vagina. Hang two Christmas ornaments from the horns and you have two festive ovaries.

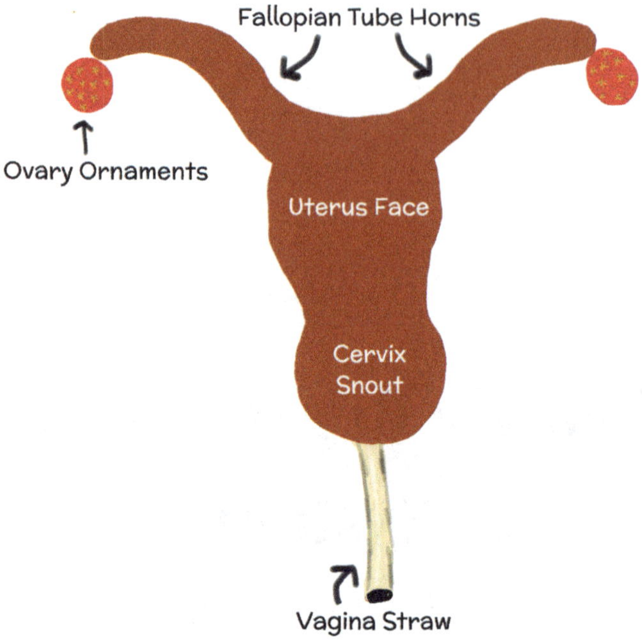

Not medically accurate.

This analogy does absolutely nothing to help explain the functionality of the system, but if you're teaching a sex ed class in the Lonestar State, it's a surefire way to remember where all the bits and pieces go.

Starting with the vagina, we're going to travel up through the cervix, into the uterus, past the fallopian tubes, and end with the ovaries. Working knowledge of female anatomy is critical to understanding everything from in vitro fertilization, to the efficacy of rape kits, to abortion itself, so don't be ashamed if you have to come back and review this section multiple times after reading other chapters.

Vaginal opening

We're not going to talk about external genitalia, a.k.a. the vulva (including the labia, clitoris, and mons pubis) because 1. It doesn't really impact the topics we'll be covering and 2. Doing so will probably get this book banned for lewd content in 48/50 states in the US. The only thing we'll touch on is the hymen, a thin membrane that partially covers the opening of the vagina. This little piece of skin has been a topic of regulation for centuries and it'll pop up again in the chapter on consent.

The vagina and pelvic floor

The vagina starts once you enter the body and does *not* include external genitalia. If someone were to kick a woman in the crotch, they'd technically be kicking them in the vulva, not the vagina. On the longhorn, this is the straw coming from the cattle's mouth. When not in use, the vaginal walls collapse inward and touch each other like an empty tube of toothpaste and because it's made of smooth muscle (not skeletal muscle) which is not under voluntary control. This means that women cannot physically open or close their reproductive tract regardless of how much they do or do not "want it."

The muscles that *are* under voluntary control are the pelvic floor muscles which extend from the bottom of the spine (coccyx) to the pubic bone. These skeletal muscles can be contracted to hold in urine or bowel movements and are sometimes strengthened with Kegel exercises in an effort to amp up a woman's sexual pleasure and/or support her internal organs.

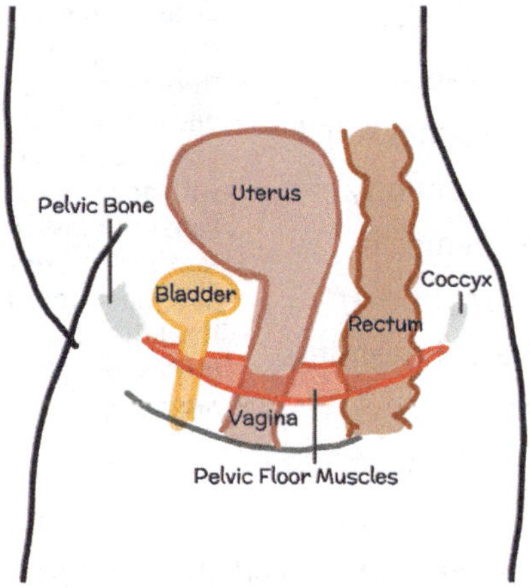

Most importantly, pelvic floor muscles help prevent a woman's uterus from falling out of her body through her vagina. Which, yes, is a thing that can happen and it's rather disturbing for the owner of the uterus when it does. During pregnancy and with age, these muscles are stretched out a bit and aside from the rare complication of uterine prolapse, this is one of the reasons many moms find themselves peeing their pants 'just a little' when they laugh too hard.

So how about that self-lubricating vag?

Turns out, that's not a thing! At least not in the way most people think it is. But it *is* a good reproductive trivia question if you ever end up at a weird party.

Vaginas are made of stratified squamous epithelium, or layers of cells. They do not have mucus producing glands anywhere in their walls. The only fluid coming directly from the vaginal walls is squeezed out from the surrounding tissue when the area becomes engorged during arousal. All the standard slippery/sticky/ever-changing secretions people think of when they think of vaginas typically come from Bartholin glands at the opening of the vagina and the cervix at the top.

Which brings us to the cervix

The 'cervix' is simply a special name for the lower portion of the uterus, the tissue of which is continuous with the vagina. You'll notice the medical community loves to give specific names to different parts of an organ even when it's all connected. Regardless of how annoying that is, it's important to understand what these words refer to if you ever read medical literature. For example, if you read a study someone referenced about whether a pregnancy complication is, or is not, deadly, you'll see descriptions like "placenta

> ***Fun fact:*** During a medical school lecture, one of my professors would add real-life tips as a reward for getting through the tedium of anatomy. During one of these add-ons he included "what to expect during a pelvic exam" with an image of a real-life cervix. I am so thankful because if I'd seen one for the first time in the wild, I would have been convinced my patient had a tiny little penis sprouting out of her uterus. Google it. I promise you, it's the most surprising image you'll see all day.

covering a portion of the cervical os". Unfortunately for regular people everywhere, very few peer-reviewed studies use layman's terms like, "meaty pregnancy organ grew over the opening of the uterus". And that's why I'll be defining a wide array of terminology throughout this book.

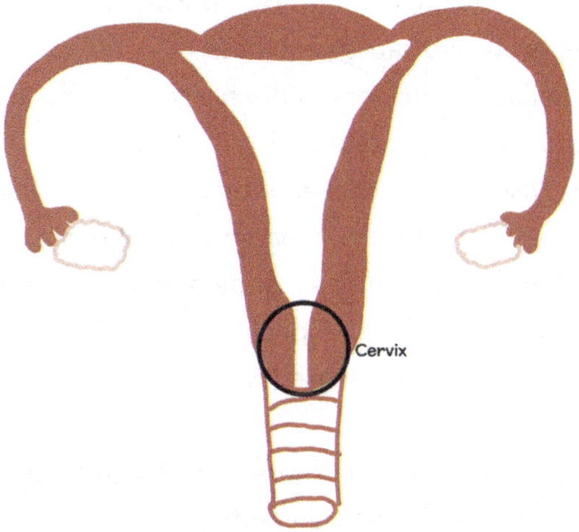

If you're looking at the longhorn diagram, the cervix is the nose. Like nostrils on a sick bull, this area secretes mucus. When a woman notices changes in the consistency and thickness of mucus she finds in her underwear throughout the month, this is the place that discharge is being created.

At the bottom of the cervix, we have the cervical os, which is just the fancy term for "cervical hole" or opening. Above the cervical os is the bottom part of the uterus, called the cervical canal. This is like the mudroom of the uterus. Everything coming in or out passes through here. In the case of child birth, the whole room expands and the doorway widens so a baby can exit. However, in any other circumstance, the doorway is a tiny pinhole and larger objects (say, the size of a penis), never enter. Small objects like sperm can wiggle through, which is good since sperm are an important part of fertilization.

Physicians view the cervix during a pelvic exam by using a speculum to open the vaginal walls and visually identify any swelling, redness, or discharge that may indicate a problem. Some common findings may include:

- White cottage-cheese-like bits could indicate a yeast infection caused by candida, a fungus that normally exists in the body, but can overgrow and cause problems.
- Foul-smelling, yellow-green discharge could be a sign of trichomoniasis, a parasitic STI.
- Thin, grayish, smelly discharge may be present in bacterial vaginosis, when there's an overgrowth of bacteria.
- Cervical motion tenderness, or pain when the cervix is moved, is an uncomfortable finding for the patient that can be a sign of Pelvic Inflammatory Disease (PID).

Identifying these problems, and others, during regular pelvic exams increases the likelihood of timely and effective treatment. Without intervention, infections of the reproductive tract, including STIs, may lead to discomfort or pain during sex, a decrease in fertility, pregnancy complications, and in some cases, cervical cancer.

On to the uterus

Now we're in the head of the cow. The uterus is a warm, magical, muscle lined room for potential babies. It's about the size of a human fist when it's unoccupied and it can stretch to the size of a watermelon, or more(!) during pregnancy. The smooth muscles lining the uterus cannot be consciously controlled, but they do clamp down with the fury of a pitbull's jaw when giving birth. On top of the smooth muscle layer (a.k.a. the myometrium) is the endometrium, a layer of tissue filled with glands and blood vessels that grows and sheds throughout the menstrual cycle.

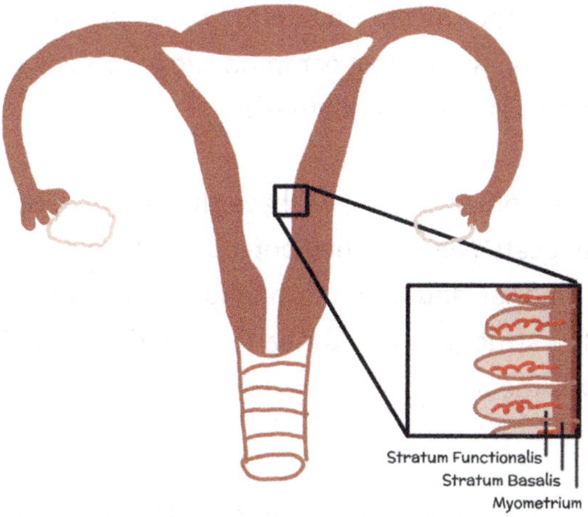

Note the two layers of the endometrium: the stratum basalis and the stratum functionalis. During a female menstrual cycle, the stratum functionalis grows and then sheds every month. The stratum basalis does not. Both layers sit on top of a thick muscular layer called the myometrium.

This is the place babies are housed, menstruation is made possible, and pregnancies go awry. It's also the inspiration for one of my favorite old-timey medical facts. In ancient Greece, philosophers believed the uterus had a mind of its own and would wander around the body causing mental health issues like hysteria.[3] When modern day politicians say something wacky about womens' bodies I like to remember this fact as proof that we have, indeed, come a long way. Even when it doesn't feel like it.

Fallopian tubes

Two hollow tubes branch off either side of the uterus and then curve downwards towards the ovaries; these are the fallopian tubes. If you were to pull one out and look at it, which you can do vicariously through anatomy dissection videos on YouTube, it would be a single tube connecting to the uterus. However, the medical powers that be gave it three sections named the isthmus (closest-to-uterus segment), the

[3] Adair, M. J. (1995). Plato's View of the "Wandering Uterus." *The Classical Journal*, *91*(2), 153–163. http://www.jstor.org/stable/3298478

ampulla (middle), and the infundibulum (closest-to-ovaries). The middle section, or ampulla, is the most common site for an egg to become fertilized as it travels towards the uterus.

At the end of the infundibulum, we have the fimbriae, or finger-like projections that catch eggs as they pop out of the ovaries once a month. Covering the fimbriae and found throughout the entire fallopian tube are tiny hair-like structures called cilia that rapidly whisk fluid from the ovaries towards the uterus.

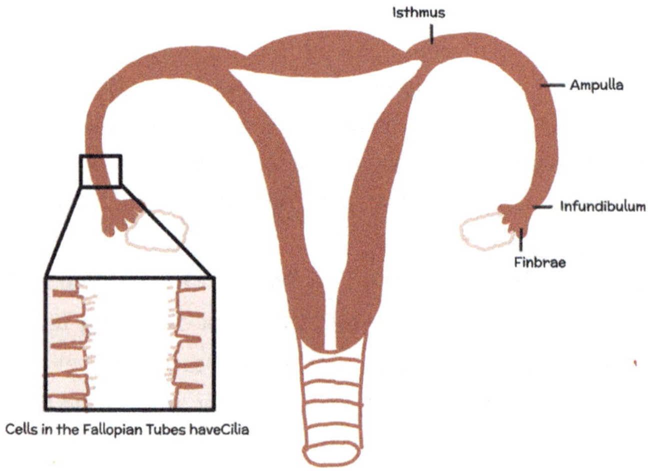

When viewed in 3D, the fimbriae aren't finger-like at all. They're more like a bouquet of folded deli meats that slowly wiggle around. However, 99% of medical textbooks refer to them as "finger-like" so I wanted to keep it consistent.

These tubes are the transportation highway for eggs and also the main site of sterilization for women who choose permanent birth control. For example, a bilateral salpingectomy removes both fallopian tubes so there's no easy path for eggs to reach the uterus, and a tubal ligation involves permanently sealing the fallopian tubes using cauterization or clips. Additionally, blockage of the fallopian tubes is a major cause of infertility because it disrupts the ability of eggs to travel from the ovaries to the uterus and also blocks sperm from reaching the eggs. Swelling or narrowing of these tubes can be caused by STIs, endometriosis (when uterine tissue grows outside of the uterus), infections and scarring.

Ovaries

Here we end our tour at the ovaries. These two oval-shaped organs at the end of the fimbriae house millions of future eggs. When a female baby is born, she'll have all the oocytes[4] she'll ever have in her little ovaries. These stores diminish as a person ages, and one (or more in some cases) will be released every month after puberty. The ovaries get interesting when we talk about conception and birth control, so we'll wait until the next chapter to go any further.

Hormones

While not technically part of the reproductive system, these chemical messengers control most of it's function post-puberty. Everything from menstruation, to mood swings, to ovulation, to menopause is dependent on tiny chemicals traveling around the body from one cell to another.

One of the most important sites for reproductive hormone release is the brain, specifically the hypothalamus and pituitary glands. The hormones from the pituitary gland are released into the bloodstream, circulate throughout the body, and then connect to receptors on cells in the reproductive system. This triggers a reaction within the cells that can influence other physical or chemical reactions. How this works will be covered in depth when we talk about ovulatory and menstrual cycles, but it's important to understand that physical anatomy isn't the only piece of the puzzle. So much of how reproduction works is down to biochemistry, and you're about to learn it all!

---

[4] Oocytes are the medical term for eggs when they are still primary or secondary follicles. You can think of these as immature eggs, but it's critical to understand that the egg released into the fallopian tubes is structurally different from the oocytes in a child's ovaries as this can sometimes complicate discussions about egg donations, birth control, and more.

What it's not

Here's a drawing of a stomach and the associated digestive system.

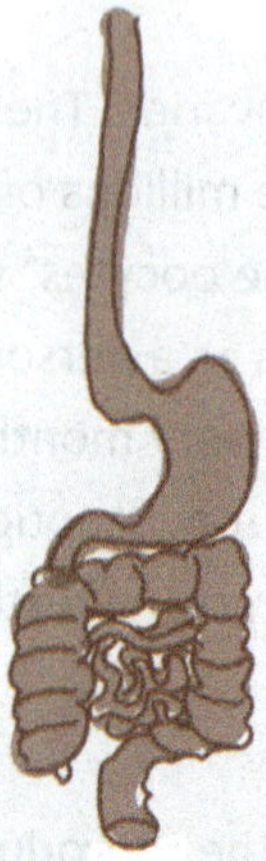

Now forget everything about this image. It has nothing to do with reproduction despite what Idaho representative, Vito Barbieri, implied when he asked if a woman could swallow a camera to see a fetus.[5] Neither a baby nor an egg ever enters this system. Unless it's a chicken egg you ate for breakfast, in which case, it will, in fact, enter your stomach.

The only exception to this rule is on a microscopic scale. The food a person consumes during pregnancy enters the digestive system where it's broken down into smaller units like proteins, lipids, carbohydrates, vitamins and other molecules. The "breaking down" part is the key phrase in that sentence. When a person takes a prenatal vitamin that's roughly the size of a full-grown donkey, it is *not* transported as a whole

[5] CBS. (2015, February 24). *Idaho lawmaker asks if swallowing small camera could allow remote gynecological exams.* CBS News. https://www.cbsnews.com/sanfrancisco/news/idaho-lawmaker-asks-if-swallowing-small-camera-could-allow-remote-gynecological-exams/

pill through the wall of the intestines and straight into the uterus where it's swallowed by the baby. It's instead broken down by enzymes in your gut so that small molecules can be absorbed into the blood through transporters in the gastrointestinal tract. Some of those molecules will be carried through the mother's bloodstream to the placenta, through the umbilical cord, and into the baby's circulation. To be clear, we're talking about things as small as vitamins (folate, B12, etc.), fatty acids, proteins, sugars (eg. glucose), the individual ingredients in certain medications, etc. Not cameras. Not sperm.[6]

More of what it's not

A person also has a urinary tract that is close to, but separate from, the reproductive system. For females, this tract starts at the base of the kidneys and exits through a completely separate hole than the vaginal entrance. Occasionally, people will suggest urinating after sex can help prevent pregnancy. Urine does not, at any point, enter the vaginal canal or reproductive system in a healthy, typical, female. However, having sex may cause bacteria and/or yeast to be pushed around the whole genital area and into the urethra due to its close proximity to the vagina. Urinating after sex might help prevent those bugs from ascending up the urethra and causing a urinary tract infection. So, pee has nothing to do with pregnancy, but it *might* help prevent UTIs.

[6] The only exception to the rule would be if a person engages in anal sex. Then, technically, there's sperm in the rectum which *is* the last part of the GI system.

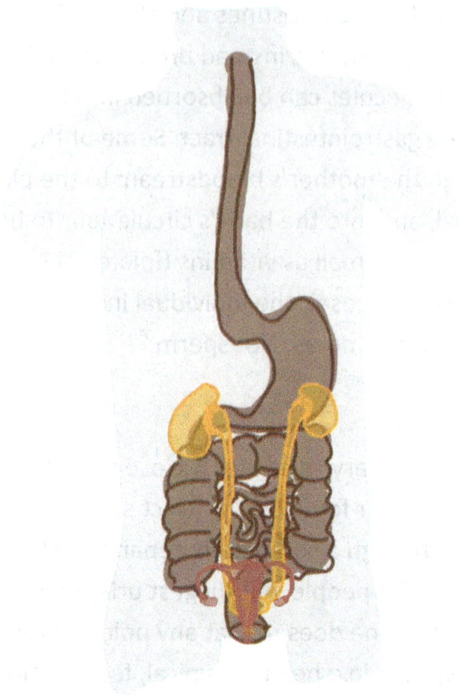

Above is an overlay of the three distinct organ systems represented by different colors. As you can see, they all live in a similar space but they never connect. Remember your anatomy and you're on your way to preventing 50%[7] of factual errors committed when arguing about abortion.

[7]I made that number up, it's completely non-factual. But, anecdotally, there's a correlation between how badly someone is made fun of on social media related to their abortion argument and how anatomically inaccurate their statement was. For example, Salt Lake County Council member, David Alvord, will never live down his tweet, "The baby is not part of the body of a woman. The umbilical chord and placenta do not directly connect to the woman. The baby floats inside the woman." Because it turns out that umbilical cords attach to placentas, and placentas attach to the uteri, and uteri are part of female bodies. The moral of the story is: Learn your anatomy. Avoid being a meme.

Chapter 2

Ovulation and Menstruation

Women are born with around 1-2 million eggs. Those eggs are then released one by one every month after puberty and are either shed during a menstrual period or become a fertilized embryo.

For the most part.

Like most things people say about female bodies, this is the middle school sex ed version and it doesn't give us enough detail when arguing about the intricacies of human ovulation and menstruation. It turns out an egg isn't just an egg. Likewise, the morning after pill alters this cycle but may not help even if you use it the morning after.

Hormones in general

Ovulation and menstruation are controlled by a series of intertwined hormones in the female body. Before we get into that, it's important to note that these hormones also exist outside of the reproductive system. Typically, before a girl has her first period (also known as menarche) she'll start to develop breasts and pubic hair. This awkward body-changing phase has a lot to do with increasing amounts of hormones like estrogens which can be released both in the ovaries once monthly ovulation starts, and in other parts of the body in non-menstruating women. Different types of estrogen can be produced in fat cells, skin cells, and even the brain![8] Peripheral production of this type of hormone is far less plentiful than what's achieved during follicular development (which we're about to cover), and after living an adult life with monthly cycles of hormone production, the decrease in sex hormones can be hard on a menopausal woman. Because of that, hormone therapy including estrogen is sometimes used to help ease symptoms of menopause like mood changes, hot flashes, vaginal dryness, and headaches. Which is a long way of saying – hormones do not exist only in one place. This chapter is going to focus on hormone production related to the reproductive system, but remember that all systems in our bodies are interconnected. While estrogen is known as a "female sex hormone," it also plays a role in cardiovascular health, bone density, and the development of certain cancers. While we won't go into the system wide effects of every hormone in this section, keep in mind that this is a very focused view of a singular part of the body.

Ovulatory Cycle

Genotypic females (humans with two X chromosomes for their 23rd pair) are typically born with 1-2 million primordial follicles.[9] These are often referred to as "eggs" by non-medical professionals, but in reality,

---

[8] Cui, J., Shen, Y., & Li, R. (2013). Estrogen synthesis and signaling pathways during aging: from periphery to brain. *Trends in molecular medicine*, *19*(3), 197–209. https://doi.org/10.1016/j.molmed.2012.12.007

[9] Duncan, F. E., Schindler, K., Schultz, R. M., Blengini, C. S., Stein, P., Stricker, S. A., Wessel, G. M., & Williams, C. J. (2020). Unscrambling the oocyte and the egg: clarifying terminology of the female gamete in mammals. *Molecular human reproduction*, *26*(11), 797–800. https://doi.org/10.1093/molehr/gaaa066

they are a specific version of the human egg at a specific phase in its lifecycle. These future eggs are diploid, meaning they still have 2 sets of chromosomes and will remain frozen in this exact phase until a person reaches puberty. During childhood and adolescence these eggs are not released and cannot be fertilized, but thousands are still lost in natural processes leaving less than half a million in the ovaries when ovulation begins.

Why does this matter?

Oral birth control and emergency contraceptive pills alter this cycle, impacting oocytes during the maturation process. Remember, oocytes are not considered "eggs" until they are released into the fallopian tubes and it's not until egg-hood that these cells are even capable of becoming fertilized. If we chemically alter the process to prevent oocytes from reaching maturation, does that become a topic of moral concern? At what point does it become ethically ambiguous – secondary follicles? Graafian follicles? Fertilized eggs? Embryos?

These topics pop up related to birth control, emergency contraceptives, IVF, and egg donation on a regular basis. I challenge you to suspend your current beliefs and allow yourself to refine your thoughts on reproductive topics from yes/no statements to "where", "when" and "how" something should, or should not, be done while reading this book.

With the start of puberty, hormone production ramps up and causes a cyclical maturation and release of an oocyte (sometimes two) every 28-40 days. This usually starts between 11-15 years old with the average age of a person's first period somewhere between 11.5 and 12.5 in the United States (between 2013-2014 the average age reported by the CDC was 11.9,[10] but that number varies by source). As this happens, a few **primordial follicles** start their natural maturation process every day, becoming **primary follicles** (also called **primary oocytes** just to complicate things). Most of these won't make it past the primary follicle phase since only one will become dominant each cycle and make it to the point of ovulation.

---

[10] Martinez GM. Trends and patterns in menarche in the United States, 1995 through 2013–2017. National Health Statistics Reports; no 146. Hyattsville, MD: National Center for Health Statistics. 2020

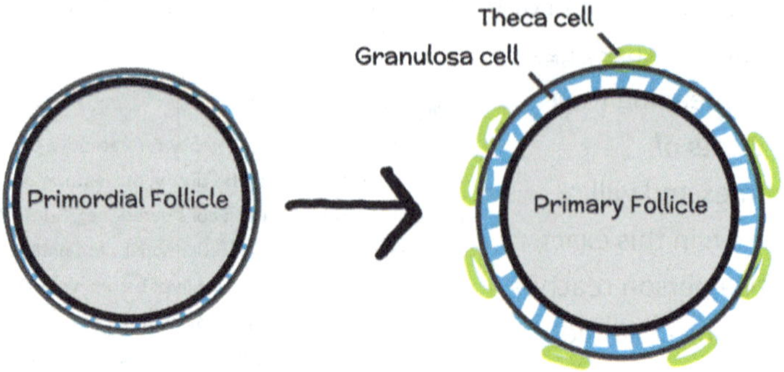

Surprisingly, this process begins not in the reproductive system at all, but in the brain. The hypothalamus produces GnRh (gonadotropin releasing hormone), which travels to the pituitary gland and stimulates the production of gonadotropins, a type of hormone that includes Follicle Stimulating Hormone (FSH) and Luteinizing Hormone (LH).

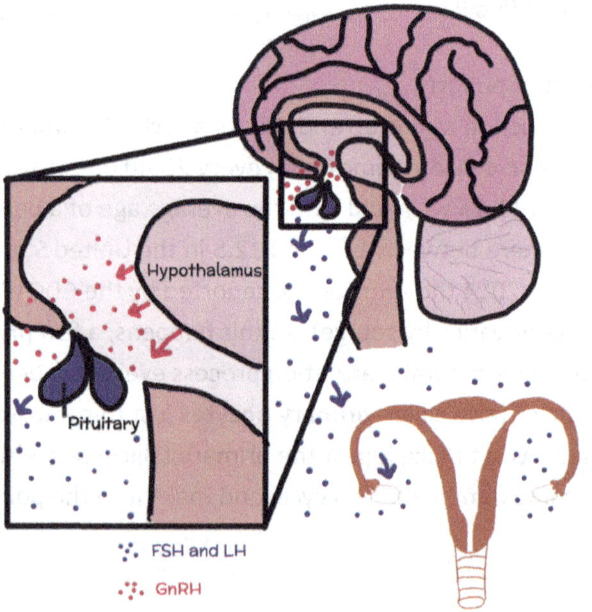

Fun observation: the pituitary gland looks like a set of testes in your brain. Easy to remember: Brain balls stimulate hormones for the reproductive cycle.

As the hypothalamus starts pumping out GnRH, it leads to FSH and LH production from the pituitary gland. Then FSH and LH stimulate a layer of cells called the zona pellucida to grow around the follicles, and around this layer of cells grows even more theca and granulosa cells.

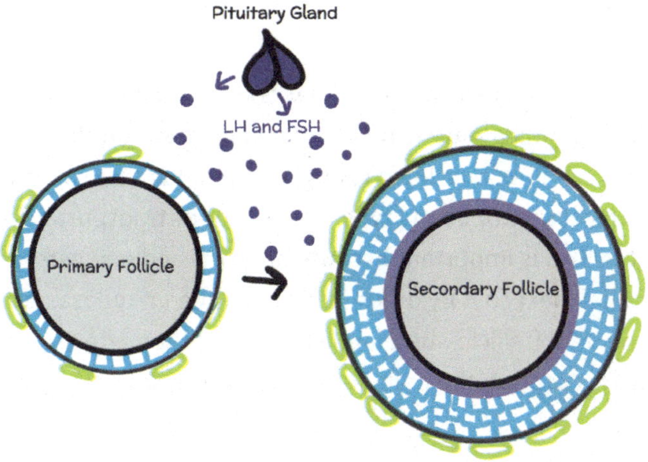

Once we have our zona pellucida, theca, and granulosa cell layers, we have a **secondary follicle**. The theca and granulosa cells are extremely important to estrogen formation and play an important role in the entire cycle.

Now this gets pretty complicated but if you're going to talk about birth control, emergency contraceptives, and/or female hormones, you need to understand some of the cells and mechanisms at play. I'll break it down to just the bits you need to know, but you'll have to stick with me to see how it all comes together at the end.

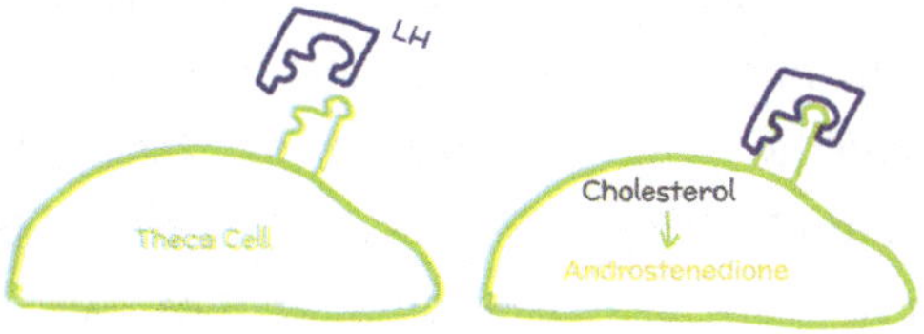

Theca cells have a receptor on them that LH (luteinizing hormone) attaches to. Think of a receptor as a puzzle piece stuck to the outside of a cell. When the matching puzzle piece floats by and attaches to it, it triggers something to happen within the cell itself. The puzzle piece floating by is the "ligand" and in the reproductive system, ligands are often hormones. When the hormone LH attaches to a receptor on theca cells, it causes cholesterol to change into an androgen hormone named androstenedione.

Androgen hormones are steroids. That doesn't mean they'll make you a competition-winning muscle builder if you increase production, it just means they are lipophilic (lipid loving) compounds that can usually diffuse into cells without any type of receptor or transporter helping them enter. This is important because androstenedione gets inside the granulosa cell next to it by diffusing through the granulosa cell's membrane. FSH (follicle-stimulating hormone) then attaches to the matching receptor on the granulosa cell and a series of events happens that causes androstenedione to eventually become estradiol (a form of estrogen).

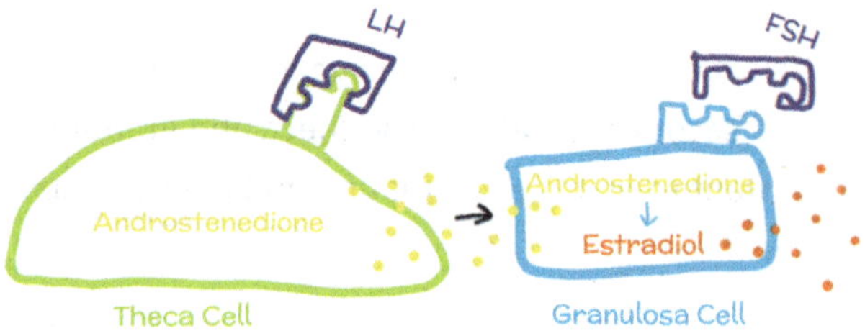

In addition to helping with estrogen creation in the granulosa cells, FSH also causes granulosa cells to start spilling out follicular fluid which slowly collects in little puddles around the follicle.

FSH continues to stimulate the oocyte over the following days, causing more estrogen to be released and follicular fluid to build up. Eventually, all the puddles of fluid connect to form one big lake called the "antrum" inside the growing clump of cells. This marks the beginning of our **tertiary follicle**, otherwise referred to as a **Graafian follicle** when fully formed. The increasing amount of estrogen released by this follicle establishes it as the dominant follicle, causing all the other follicles to give up and die off mid-maturation. As you can see, oocytes are lost at nearly every stage throughout the month, not just the one that becomes dominant and is eventually released during ovulation.

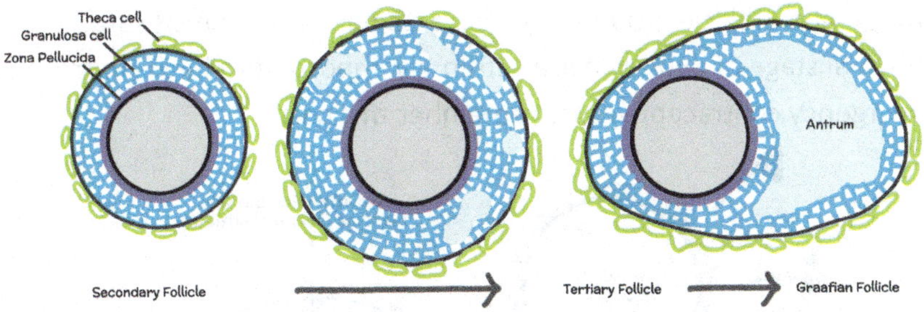

To summarize: LH production *in the brain* causes cells on a primary follicle/oocyte *in the ovary* to produce an androgen hormone. That hormone is used by the granulosa cells on the same follicle/oocyte to make estradiol (estrogen) when stimulated by FSH. This all leads up to a single follicle/oocyte growing into a Graafian follicle, and all other growing follicles/oocytes die off.

During this time the pituitary gland is still releasing FSH, and FSH is still stimulating granulosa cells which leads to more estrogen creation. Estrogen builds up until about day 12 of a cycle when it peaks.

And here's where things get truly complicated. If you remember, GnRH is released by the hypothalamus and causes the pituitary gland to release FSH and LH. When GnRH is squeezed out at a lower pulse frequency, it stimulates more FSH than LH.[11] This is one of the reasons why FSH levels are higher in the beginning of an ovulatory cycle. While the first half of the follicular phase is dominated by FSH, estrogen released from the dominant follicle is the main hormone during the second half. Estrogen reaches a tipping point and the peak levels are sensed by the hypothalamus which starts pumping out GnRH at a higher frequency. This triggers the pituitary gland to produce a huge LH surge.

---

[11] Holesh JE, Bass AN, Lord M. Physiology, Ovulation. [Updated 2023 May 1]. In: StatPearls [Internet]. Treasure Island (FL): StatPearls Publishing; 2023 Jan-. Available from: https://www.ncbi.nlm.nih.gov/books/NBK441996/

This surge happens for 36-48 hours and causes the oocyte to pop out of the Graafian follicle around day 14 in a 28 day cycle. The LH surge and the final stage of ovulation are extremely important to birth control and emergency contraceptives, so remember this part.

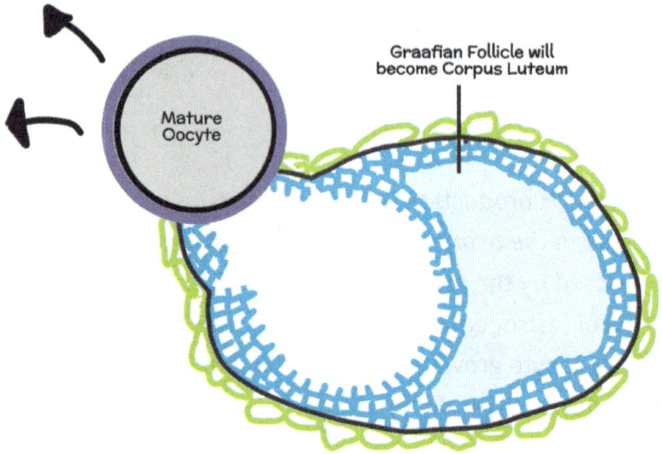

Welcome to ovulation!

Out pops the **mature oocyte**, which we can now refer to as an "egg". The oocyte/egg (even when a part of the primary follicle, secondary follicle, and Graafian follicle) still has two sets of chromosomes and will not become haploid (meaning 23 instead of 46 chromosomes) unless a sperm fertilizes it.

At this point, the fimbriae on the end of the fallopian tubes are sweeping along the ovaries so they can grab the egg as soon as it's released. From there, it's carried onwards by little hairs called "cilia" lining the fallopian tubes.

Left behind in the ovary is a blob of cells that once made up the Graafian follicle. This lump of cells is now the **corpus luteum** and will hang out for another 10-14 days if the egg is not fertilized. Don't forget about this guy; he'll be important when we talk about what's happening in the uterus during this time.

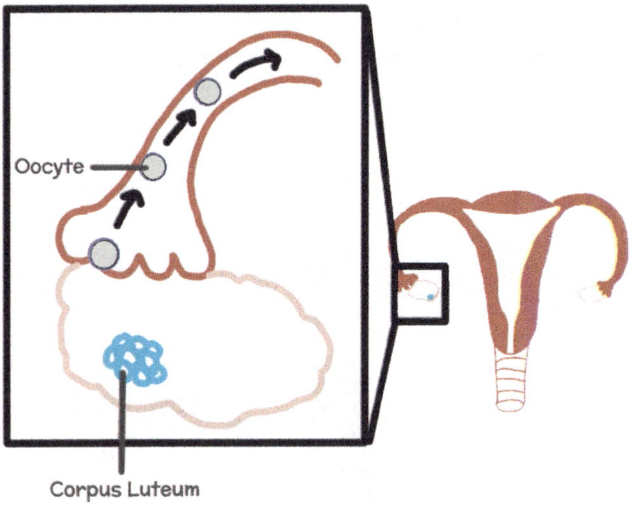

To put this all in an easily digestible format, see the example below. Every woman is slightly different so you should assume throughout this book that any time-related reference for female cycles or fetal development is approximate. This is designed as a helpful tool to wrap your head around what's going on at any given time, not a rigid calendar.

Day 1 - Hypothalamus is releasing GnRH. GnRH tells the pituitary to release FSH and LH which increase during the follicular phase.

Day 1-7 - FSH is the dominant hormone in the early follicular phase. By binding to FSH receptors on granulosa cells, it stimulates the conversion of androgens to estrogen and leads to the increase of follicular fluid.

Day 12-13 - Estrogen accumulates because the granulosa cells are releasing more and more. Once estrogen peaks, it helps trigger the LH surge.

Day 14 - LH surge causes ovulation.

Day 15 - After ovulation, FSH and LH drop dramatically.

Day 15-28 - The corpus luteum produces progesterone. If an egg is not fertilized, the corpus luteum will disintegrate and stop producing progesterone around day 28. If a pregnancy occurs, the corpus luteum will continue to help with hormone production until the placenta takes over.

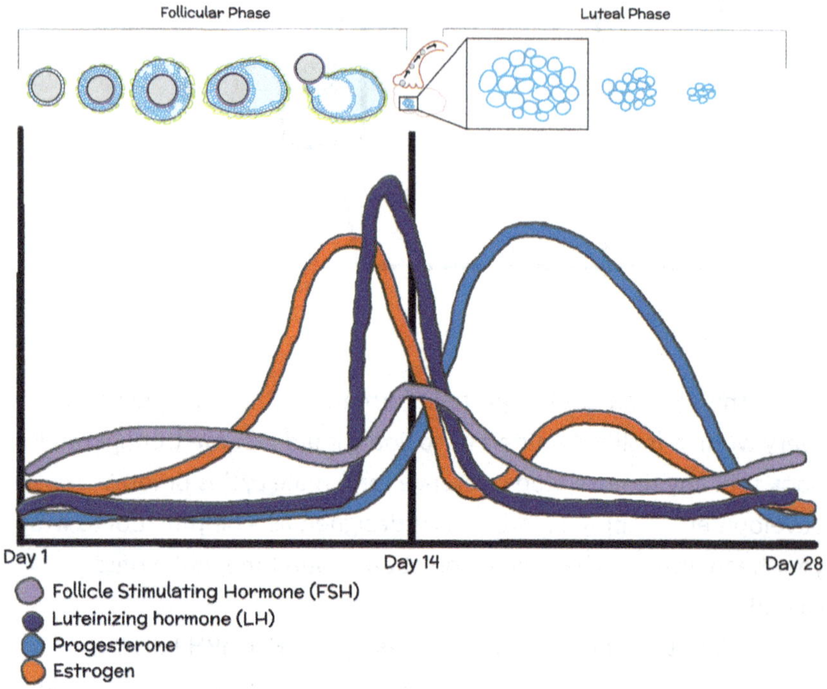

The LH surge is incredibly important in IVF, egg donation, emergency contraceptive pills, and natural family planning.

While this is all happening in the ovaries, a totally different cycle is happening in the uterus and when it comes to any type of medical intervention you'll need to have a firm grasp of both regions, so let's take a look at the menstrual cycle.

Menstrual Cycle

This is all about the uterus. Unfortunately, for those of you who prefer not to think about monthly periods, it's time to acknowledge them. The menstrual cycle fills in the gap between when an egg is released and when pregnancy might (or might not) happen. It's integral to our understanding of hormonal and emergency contraceptives.

Go back to the single oocyte that popped out of the Graafian follicle around day 14 of the ovulatory cycle. Two things are about to happen:

In the ovaries day 14-28(ish): The Graafian follicle is left behind and becomes a lump of cells called the "corpus luteum". The corpus luteum will produce a lot of progesterone and a little bit of estrogen. Assuming pregnancy does not occur, this will last for about 14 days with peak progesterone production in the middle, right before it starts to wither away. In the ovaries, this is called the **luteal phase** (corpus LUTEUM = luteal phase) and is dominated by progesterone production.

Around the same time in the uterus day 15-28(ish): While the corpus luteum is pumping out progesterone in the ovary, the uterus has entered the **secretory phase**. Progesterone hormones will attach to progesterone receptors (Pgr) on cells in the uterine cavity.[12] Remember, receptors are similar to little puzzle pieces stuck on the outside of cells that connect to their matching pieces (a.k.a. ligands). This binding triggers something to happen inside the cell. When progesterone fits into a Pgr receptor, the end result is the thickening of the top layer, or stratum functionalis, of the endometrial lining.

---

[12]Lee, K., Jeong, J., Tsai, M. J., Tsai, S., Lydon, J. P., & DeMayo, F. J. (2006). Molecular mechanisms involved in progesterone receptor regulation of uterine function. *The Journal of steroid biochemistry and molecular biology, 102*(1-5), 41–50. https://doi.org/10.1016/j.jsbmb.2006.09.006

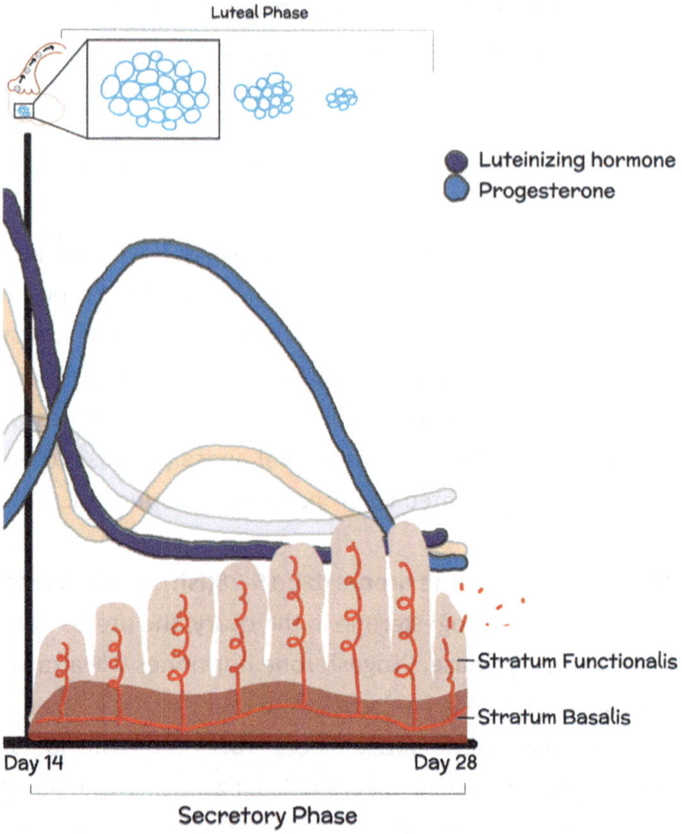

If you were to scoop out a bit of endometrium during the secretory phase and examine it under a microscope, it would be about 5 mm thick, the thickest it gets in an average menstrual cycle. You would also see lots of little coiled arteries delivering blood and nutrients to the thick endometrial tissue. Inside the uterine cavity you'd find increased secretions, hence the name "secretory phase," making a broth of fluids including glycogen, lipids, and proteins that make the uterus ripe for implantation. Think of it like a baby-friendly soup.

Lower down in the cervix, thicker mucus eventually creates a plug, preventing unwanted substances from entering the uterus like bacteria and/or additional sperm. Extra immune cells also start to gather in the uterus to keep it a healthy, safe environment for a future fetus. If an egg is fertilized during this time, it will attempt to implant into the thick, juicy endometrial wall where the environment is prime for baby-growing thanks to the effects of progesterone.

For now, let's assume fertilization does *not* happen. The egg will enter the uterus, fail to attach, and both the egg and the corpus luteum will deteriorate.

With the end of the corpus luteum comes the end of the luteal phase. With its demise, progesterone levels plummet, causing menstruation (typically day 1-5 of a cycle).

Imagine a friend tells you it's about time for her period to start and she's feeling exhausted. Her belly is unusually fluffy, her boobs are sore, her mood is all over the place, and she's nauseous (but simultaneously fighting the urge to eat chocolate covered potato chips). What would you guess is going on?
She's pregnant, right?
Actually, probably not, unless she specifically started the conversation with "I had a ton of unprotected sex this month..."

In data pulled from a popular menstrual tracking app, the following symptoms were logged by users in the days before menstruation: fatigue (85% of survey respondents), bloating (81%), tender breasts (74%), mood swings (73%), cravings (71%), and nausea (65%). These premenstrual syndrome (PMS) symptoms may be caused by an increased sensitivity to progesterone and estrogen levels during the the luteal phase, especially as progesterone suddenly drops when the corpus luteum deteriorates. Hormonal birth control may help control symptoms of PMS and it's more severe cousin, PMDD, by keeping levels steady with a progesterone lookalike, progestin. Keeping levels steady prevents the massive withdrawal.

Question to ponder:
Pregnancy is counted from a woman's last period, not the date of fertilization. Therefore if a person becomes pregnant, their first missed period will mark week 4 of pregnancy. Considering PMS symptoms so heavily overlap those of early pregnancy, would you be able to recognize the difference in the first week or two?

Ponzo, S., Wickham, A., Bamford, R., Radovic, T., Zhaunova, L., Peven, K., Klepchukova, A., & Payne, J. L. (2022). *Menstrual cycle-associated symptoms and workplace productivity in US employees: A cross-sectional survey of users of the Flo mobile phone app*. Digital health, 8, 20552076221145852. https://doi.org/10.1177/20552076221145852

No more progesterone leads to the following:

- No more cell proliferation in the uterus (the stratum functionalis stops growing)
- Less control of the coiled blood vessels in the stratum functionalis causing them to dilate and constrict until they burst
- Immune cell concentration decreases in uterus
- Loss of thickened mucus plug in the cervix
- Increased production of GnRH by the hypothalamus

Put it all together and we have the coiled arteries in the endometrium contracting (tightening) and dilating (loosening) until eventually these small blood vessels in the stratum functionalis weaken to the point they burst. Pools of blood build up in the endometrium as the broken arteries leak, interrupting the blood supply to the top layer of cells. Lack of blood means death, causing the top layer to slough off. The resulting bloody mix of dead cells slides out through the cervix and into the vagina when the mucus plug thins.

> **Question to ponder:** Does your state exempt period products from taxation. Do high schools in your region provide free feminine hygiene products? If not, would you support legislation to do so?
> A woman spends, on average, $1,800 over a lifetime on pads and tampons alone. This does not cover additional period related costs like pain relief meds for menstrual cramps, replacement clothing when pads and tampons leak, and/or lost work wages from PMS/PMDD symptoms. To offset the financial burden of menstruation, 25 states exempt pads and tampons from sales tax as of June 2023. Additionally, states including Illinois, New Hampshire, New York, Virginia, and Washington, require schools to provide period products to menstruating students.
>
> Rodriguez, L. (2021, October 1). 20 places around the world where governments provide free period products. Global Citizen. https://www.globalcitizen.org/en/content/free-period-products-countries-cities-worldwide/

And this, my friends, is "the period". Starting at menarche and continuing until her 40s or 50s, an average American woman will spend about 3,500 days of her life menstruating. During that time she'll use around 17,000 tampons or pads.[13], costing about $1,800 total.

[13] Berg, S. (2020, December 16). *Why stigma prevents treating menstrual hygiene as essential.* American Medical Association.

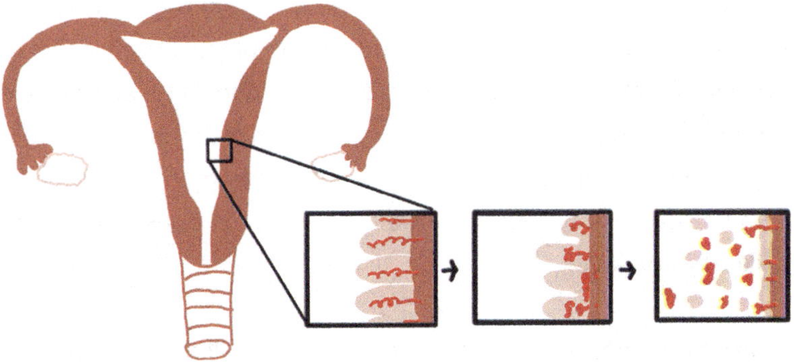

The end of menstruation signals the start of the **proliferative** phase in the uterus, causing the whole cycle to restart. Let's refer back to our diagram to see what's happening in the ovaries at this point.

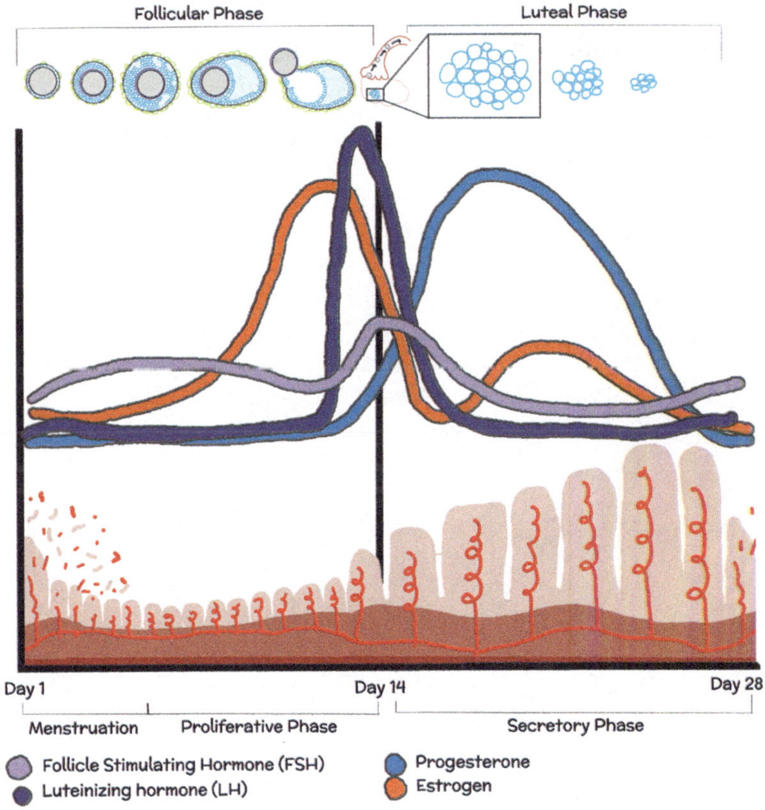

---

https://www.ama-assn.org/delivering-care/population-care/why-stigma-prevents-treating-menstrual-hygiene-essential

The estrogen that's created by the granulosa cells in the ovaries will cause the proliferative stage to continue in the uterus. During this time, the stratum functionalis will regenerate slowly and spiral arteries will grow between days 6-14 (side note: How cool is it that people's bodies grow a whole network of new blood vessels every month?). Notice the stratum basalis, or lower layer of the uterine lining, does not change or shed like the top layer.

Right around ovulation, the mucus in the cervix will thin enough for sperm to easily pass into the uterus searching for eggs to fertilize. When ovulation happens around day 14, the mucus thickens up again and we start all over at the beginning of the chapter.

Over and over until menopause.

Chapter 3

Altering the Cycle

If you think you already know enough to argue like a doc' about how medications can impact hormonal cycles, give the following questions a try before skipping ahead:

1. What steroid hormone is released by the corpus luteum and can maintain early pregnancy?

2. What hormone analogs (lookalikes) can be used as a monthly contraceptive pill *and* emergency contraceptives?

3. Medications containing what class of hormone can be used to treat symptoms of uterine fibroids, polycystic ovarian syndrome, and may also help prevent ovarian and endometrial cancer?

Answers:

1. Progesterone
2. Progestins
3. Progestogens

Do those all sound alike to you? Progesterone is a steroid hormone produced naturally by the corpus luteum and placenta to help maintain pregnancy. Progestins are synthetic versions of progesterone that include drugs like Levonorgestrel and norgestrel, found in both monthly birth control and emergency contraceptive pills. Both progesterone and progestins fall under the larger category of progestogens.

How'd you do? Don't worry, most people get at least one wrong. If you happen to be "most people" the bad news is, you have learning to do. The good news is, you'll soon be winning arguments against all the people who don't do the learning!

I once tried hormonal birth control when I was 20-something years old. Within a month, my boobs blew up like balloons, zits erupted across my face like a chain of volcanoes, and my midsection burst forth from my waistband like a sausage that had been hopelessly overstuffed. After commiserating with a friend of mine, she explained: "You know the pill just tricks your body into thinking it's pregnant". That checked out based on personal experience considering that when I got pregnant I had the same set of discomforts.

And this is why anecdotal evidence alone is not a good basis for medical understanding.

Let's take a look at what's *really* happening when someone takes birth control pills.

Oral contraceptives come in two flavors: progestin only and progestin plus a synthetic estrogen. Progestins are progesterone analogs, meaning chemically, they look and act like the real thing. Because they look similar, progestins can bind to the same receptors that progesterone normally would, tricking your body into thinking progesterone levels are elevated. And while it's true that progesterone levels skyrocket during pregnancy, the synthetic stuff is given at doses that only elevate levels a little bit; much closer to where we would see progesterone immediately after ovulation.

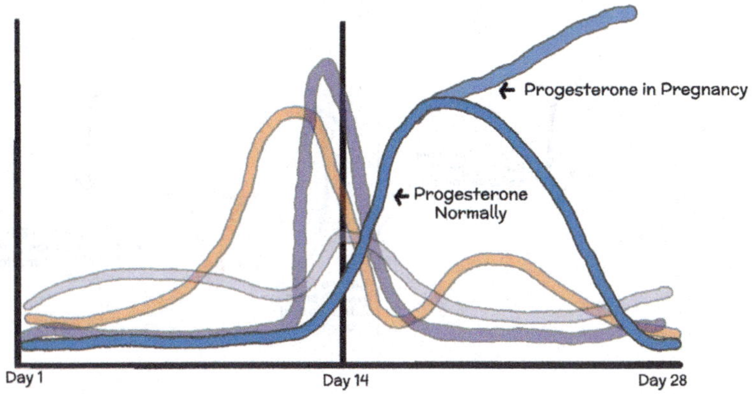

Typically, progesterone levels increase when an egg is released thanks to the remaining corpus luteum in the ovary. During that time, the body does *not* want another oocyte to develop since it's waiting to see if the one that was just released will be fertilized or not. If fertilization happens, the body needs to funnel all its resources to the growing embryo, meaning any more effort spent maturing more follicles would be a huge waste of time and energy. Progesterone from the corpus luteum also slows down the hypothalamus' production of GnRH. Less GnRH means less stimulation for the pituitary gland, causing less production of FSH and LH.[14]

---

[14] Cooper DB, Patel P, Mahdy H. Oral Contraceptive Pills. [Updated 2022 Nov 24]. In: StatPearls [Internet]. Treasure Island (FL): StatPearls Publishing; 2023 Jan-. Available from: https://www.ncbi.nlm.nih.gov/books/NBK430882/

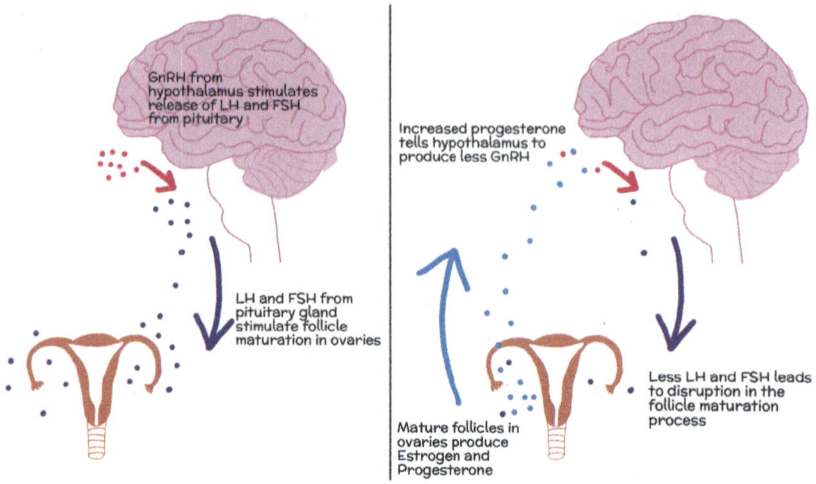

In short, increased progesterone in a normal cycle signals to the brain that ovulation just happened. If a body just ovulated, it doesn't want to restart the oocyte maturation process until it knows a pregnancy has failed to occur. Why waste the resources?

If progesterone is artificially elevated with oral birth control pills (similar to levels seen after ovulation), the same thing happens. The artificial progestins will decrease the amount of GnRH, which reduces FSH and LH. Additionally, because follicles are not maturing, they are not producing their own estrogen. Estrogen helps stimulate the mid-cycle LH surge so without it reaching peak levels, the surge will not occur.

Less maturation of follicles, no LH surge, no ovulation.

If we allow things to progress normally, the corpus luteum falls apart when the egg is not fertilized and there's a huge drop in progesterone. That drop signals that there's no baby, and it's time for the body to start funneling resources to develop another oocyte. After all, humans are just a bunch of animals with a biological need to perpetuate our own species so our reproductive systems will constantly work towards that goal.

If a person is on birth control, it's safe to assume they do *not* want more oocytes to develop. Mature eggs mean the possibility of pregnancy. We prevent this by keeping progesterone levels higher for longer so you won't see the same rise and drop in progesterone at the same time you normally would.

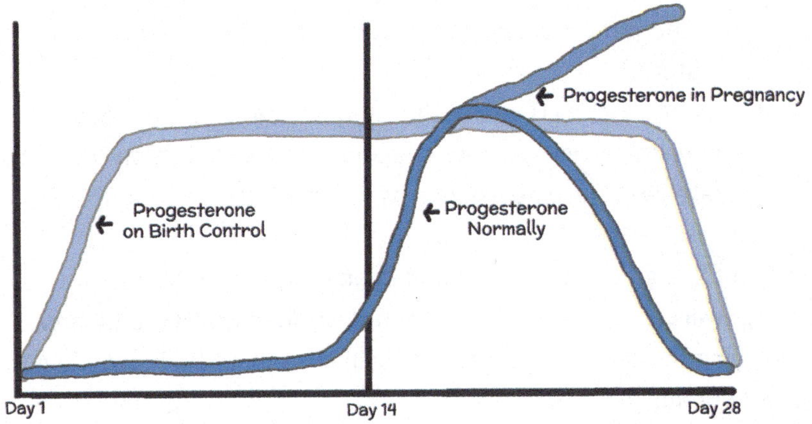

However, if a person is taking oral birth control and still chooses to have a period, she'll need to stop putting progestin into her body for a period of time triggering menstruation. To do this, a person takes the "inactive" pills in their oral BC dispenser for several days. Depending on the brand, women can menstruate as often as once a month or as infrequently as 4 times a year. Remember, hormonal birth control keeps progesterone stimulation relatively even; the stratum functionalis is not triggered to start proliferating in the same way it would naturally. Although it *does* grow, it doesn't become as thick and juicy as it would during an unaltered cycle. Because of that, people using birth control may have lighter periods when they do have them (less tissue = less gunk to lose), and there's not much harm in avoiding menstruation because the endometrial lining isn't getting massive like it would during a natural secretory phase.

To summarize: When you introduce progestin pills into the cycle, the drop in progesterone doesn't happen in the same way at the same time.

This tricks the body into behaving like ovulation just occurred for longer than usual and the following things happen:

1. The hypothalamus will keep the brakes on GnRH production (just like it would when the corpus luteum is producing progesterone).
2. This decrease prevents LH and FSH from reaching higher levels.
3. Without the increase in FSH stimulation, follicles never fully mature.
4. A decrease in LH means the all-important LH surge doesn't happen, so neither does ovulation. Lack of ovulation is the key takeaway since no egg means no possible fertilization.

Pills containing both progestins and ethinyl estradiol (an estrogen analog) will cause an even greater suppression of GnRH production, amplifying this effect. However, estrogen analogs on their own do not prevent pregnancy.

Fun fact: when using hormonal birth control pills the cervical mucus thickens just like it does around day 14 of a normal cycle. With progestin-containing pills, the thickening of cervical mucus is almost immediate, with mucosal changes peaking 3-4 hours after taking a pill. This mucous block can remain nearly impenetrable to sperm for up to 22-24 hours, stopping sperm from ever entering the cervical canal in the first place.[15] This is double protection: no ovulation + no sperm entry!

To revisit my friend's claim: Does birth control trick a body into being pregnant? No, not really. While not entirely accurate, it's more like tricking your body into thinking ovulation just occurred. Either way, the main mechanism of action here is preventing an egg from maturing and

---

[15] Han, L., Padua, E., Hart, K. D., Edelman, A., & Jensen, J. T. (2019). Comparing cervical mucus changes in response to an oral progestin or oestrogen withdrawal in ovarian-suppressed women: a clinical pilot. *The European journal of contraception & reproductive health care : the official journal of the European Society of Contraception*, *24*(3), 209–215. https://doi.org/10.1080/13625187.2019.1605503

being released. If we don't have an oocyte enter the fallopian tubes, we don't have the potential for pregnancy which is why birth control pills are reported to be 99% effective if taken correctly.

Real world efficacy

But wait! 99% efficacy is based on lab studies of progestin and it turns out lab results do not equal real world efficacy. Like most medications, there's a difference between the expected and actual results. Why? In a human body, there are hundreds of cell types, thousands of receptors on those cells, millions of possible chemical interactions, and such a staggering degree of variation, science has hardly scratched the surface of what you can expect when introducing different drugs to different people at different doses.

In the case of hormonal contraception, there's another big factor that alters effectiveness more than anything else: consistency of use. Oral contraceptives require users to take a pill every 24 hours for full pregnancy-preventing effects. If someone has a meeting that runs late and forgets their pill at home? There's only a three hour window before efficacy starts to wane. The more often a person delays or skips a dose, the less effective coverage will be that month. Combine that with all the other complexities of a human body and oral birth control comes in at a real-world efficacy rate of about 91% according to the American College of Obstetricians and Gynecologists (ACOG). That means that if 100 women use oral contraceptives over the course of a year, 9 will still get pregnant.

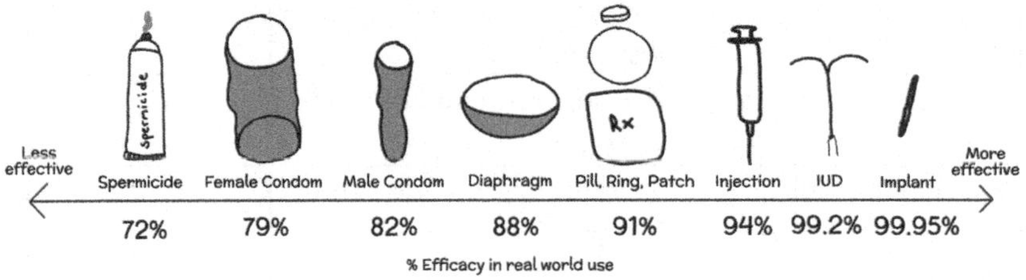

Modern medicine tries to combat this gap in efficacy by offering up additional routes of administration. Transdermal patches can be stuck to a person's skin like a band-aid and only need to be changed once a week. Vaginal rings are inserted into the vagina and left right below the cervix for a month at a time. While they're good options for patients who can't remember to take a pill, both still have a 9% fail rate.

There's a small jump in efficacy to 94% (6% fail rate) when we inject progestins every three months. User error is nearly eliminated for three months at a time since it's based on a single shot. The next big jump in efficacy that nearly matches the 99%+ claim of progestin containing birth control is seen with an implant like Nexplanon, a tiny rod slowly releases progestin into a person's arm for up to three years without any follow-up action needed.

Birth control type and brand name	**Hormones contained**	**Real world efficacy based on type**
Nexplanon, implant	Etonogestrel (an estrogen)	99.9%
Depo-Provera, injection	Medroxyprogesterone acetate (a progestin)	94%
Xulane, transdermal patch	Norelgestromin (a progestin) and ethinyl estradiol (an estrogen)	91%
Twirla, transdermal patch	Levonorgestrel (a progestin) and ethinyl estradiol	91%
Annovera, vaginal ring	Segesterone acetate (a progestin) and ethinyl estradiol	91%
Nuvaring, vaginal ring	Etonogestrel and ethinyl estradiol	91%
Amethia and Jolessa, combined birth control pill	Levonorgestrel and ethinyl estradiol	91%

Yaz, combined birth control pill	Drospirenone (a progestin) and ethinylestradiol	91%
Camila, Errin, and Jolivette, mini-pill	Norethindrone (a progestin)	91%

Access to contraceptives

Even if we're working with a 6% fail rate, having more than a 90% chance of preventing pregnancy sounds pretty good compared to the mere 82% of pregnancies prevented with condoms. As abortion regulations tighten, more women are considering turning to oral contraceptives so they don't end up in a situation they don't want to be in.

Despite birth control being legal since 1972, access to contraceptives is constantly in flux due to health insurance regulations. For example, the American Care Act (a.k.a. the ACA, a.k.a. Obamacare) mandated coverage for hormonal contraceptives with no out-of-pocket expense. However, in July, 2020 the Trump administration ruled that employers could decline contraception coverage on religious grounds despite national insurance regulations. Once again, in January, 2023 Biden's team introduced a new stipulation, not yet passed as of June '23, that would reverse the religious exemption by stating all insurance plans governed by the ACA would be required to offer contraceptives at no cost regardless of religious beliefs.

Question to ponder: Knowing what you now know about the mechanics of hormonal birth control pills, would you consider its use a violation of your religious beliefs? As a thought exercise, would you consider birth control a violation of *any* religious beliefs? Can you back up that argument, whatever it may be, with your newfound medical understanding?

The back and forth is exhausting and it means there's still plenty of room left for debate. It also means that as I'm writing this, people who get their insurance through religious organizations may not have access to hormonal contraceptives.

Allowing religious organizations to decline contraceptive coverage is one thing. But what happens when those regulations impact patients who use contraceptives for non-sex-related purposes? For example, Polycystic Ovarian Syndrome (PCOS) is a complex syndrome that can cause serious complications including extremely heavy, painful menstrual periods and infertility. In PCOS, many follicles form in the ovaries simultaneously and cause an increase in ovarian diameter which can lead to pelvic pain and interruptions in ovulation. Externally, people who have PCOS may have increased body hair, loss of head-hair, and excessive, painful acne. According to the American Academy of Family Physicians (AAFP), oral contraceptives are considered a first-line treatment for PCOS symptoms including dysmenorrhea (painful periods) and irregular menstrual cycles.[16]

Should religious exemptions that allow organizations to refuse coverage for contraceptives also allow coverage to be denied to young girls who suffer from extreme monthly pain? If not, what is the criteria separating medical necessity from contraceptive use? This is a problem we'll see pop up time and again with medication regulation. How do you differentiation between use case and who draws this sometimes arbitrary line?

On the flip side, if religious insurance providers were forced to cover contraceptives for medically necessary use but not contraceptive use, what happens if a sexually active young girl wants birth control to prevent pregnancy and complains of dysmenorrhea (painful periods) to get it covered as a non-contraceptive?

If you thought birth control wasn't relevant anymore, these questions demonstrate just how much the conversation still matters.

---

[16] Williams, T., Mortada, R., & Porter, S. (2016). Diagnosis and Treatment of Polycystic Ovary Syndrome. *American family physician*, *94*(2), 106–113.

And if we take a step back from the gray area of use case, should religious organizations even have a problem with hormonal contraceptives since they don't impact fertilized eggs or end a pregnancy?

I don't have an answer, but if you're someone who defends universal coverage of contraceptives (or, on the other side, religious exemption), *you* should. These are questions that should be asked of any regulator who proposes we deny healthcare coverage of any medication approved for use in the United States. Alternatively, people who argue against religious exemptions should also have a deep understanding of *why* they feel that way, backed up by medical facts.

Now, consider the fact that progestin analogs and progesterone are used for portions of IVF cycles, amenorrhea (the absence of menstruation), dysregulated menstrual cycles, premature ovarian failure, Turner syndrome, menopause, hypogonadism, and preventing miscarriage.[17] In which of these cases should religious organizations be able to deny medical coverage? In which should they be forced to comply?

What about the plethora of non-contraceptive medications that alter the ovulatory or menstrual cycles, occasionally leading to a lack of ovulation just like birth control? For example, non-steroidal anti-inflammatory drugs (NSAIDs) commonly used to treat rheumatoid arthritis symptoms can prevent ovulation in 75%-93% of women depending on the dose. These drugs include meloxicam, diclofenac,

---

[17] Edwards M, Can AS. Progestin. [Updated 2023 Mar 11]. In: StatPearls [Internet]. Treasure Island (FL): StatPearls Publishing; 2023 Jan-. Available from: https://www.ncbi.nlm.nih.gov/books/NBK563211/

naproxen and etoricoxib[18] [19] With over 90% efficacy in preventing ovulation, diclofenac is almost as effective of a contraceptive as progestin. Should this justify a religious organization denying coverage of a medication like diclofenac sodium/misoprostol to someone suffering from rheumatoid arthritis?

And if insurance coverage of hormonal contraceptives is denied, shouldn't there be an effective alternative for women who want to choose when they start a family?

---

[18] Jesam, C., Salvatierra, A. M., Schwartz, J. L., Fuentes, A., & Croxatto, H. B. (2014). Effect of oral administration of a continuous 18 day regimen of meloxicam on ovulation: experience of a randomized controlled trial. *Contraception*, *90*(2), 168–173. https://doi.org/10.1016/j.contraception.2014.04.011

[19] European League Against Rheumatism. (2015, June 11). Non-steroidal anti-inflammatory drugs inhibit ovulation after just 10 days. *ScienceDaily*. Retrieved June 21, 2023 from www.sciencedaily.com/releases/2015/06/150611082124.htm

Chapter 4

Non-Medical Contraception & the myth of preventable pregnancy

The implication that a person *chose* to get pregnant looms over nearly every modern discussion about abortion, childcare, education, and parental rights. However, we saw that even with one of the most common forms of contraception, the hormonal contraceptive pill, there's a 9% fail rate. If a person uses condoms, that jumps to 18%.

Even outside of birth control failure rates, the idea of pregnancy as a "preventable" condition has a host of practical issues. Technically, in the case of abstinence, it is preventable.[20] However, that's not a realistic

[20] The exception being survivors of sexual assault who have all choices, including abstinence, stolen from them through no fault of their own.

option for many women. Sexual intercourse can be considered a martial responsibility, especially in marriage. It's a cornerstone of "duty" in many a religious union (and not just Christianity, although I'm quoting the Bible below).

> *But since sexual immorality is occurring, each man should have sexual relations with his own wife, and each woman with her own husband. The husband should fulfill his marital duty to his wife, and likewise the wife to her husband.* ***The wife does not have authority over her own body but yields it to her husband****. In the same way, the husband does not have authority over his own body but yields it to his wife.* ***Do not deprive each other*** *except perhaps by mutual consent and for a time, so that you may devote yourselves to prayer. Then come together again so that Satan will not tempt you because of your lack of self-control.*
>
> *1 Corinthians 7:2-5*

Don't see how that's important? 46 out of every 1,000 pregnancies in married women are aborted.[21] This makes sense if someone is religiously or culturally bound to provide sex in her marriage and the majority of birth control is not 100% effective.

As an alternative to medical contraception, fertility apps like Natural Cycles, an FDA approved Natural Family Planning (NFP) tracker, have been popping up in discussions as reliable solutions.

Natural Family Planning (NFP) advocates occasionally offer up NFP as a birth control alternative that can be used when healthcare coverage for oral contraceptives isn't available. You may have seen it promoted by the Catholic Church due to their historically anti-contraceptive stance. In the "Vademecum for confessors concerning some aspects of the

[21] Kortsmit K, Nguyen AT, Mandel MG, et al. Abortion Surveillance — United States, 2020. MMWR Surveill Summ 2022;71(No. SS-10):1–27. DOI: http://dx.doi.org/10.15585/mmwr.ss7110a1

morality of conjugal life" presentation by the Vatican, this was made clear with the reference to the "objective evil of contraception."[22] Logically, the church would promote a natural alternative considering almost every religious organization recognizes that not all families, at all times, are ready to start or continue having children.

NFP, used for religious or non-religious purposes, is a method of tracking body temperature, cervical secretions and dates of menstruation to identify fertile and non-fertile periods. Based on what we learned about ovulatory and menstrual cycles, this should be easy, right? During fertile times, a woman may choose to use a barrier contraceptive or abstain from sex all together if she'd like to prevent pregnancy. In theory, this is a great idea and some studies show less than a 2% fail rate with typical use and less than a 1% failure with perfect use.[23] That's better than condoms, birth control pills, and injections!

However, there are equally reliable studies that show a 25% fail rate. One in four women using NFP will end up pregnant within a year.

Now imagine this seemingly unrelated scenario. A room full of anthrax. When inhaled, it has an 80% chance of killing you.[24] In a hypothetical scenario, scientists invent a new respiratory device that protects against

---

[22] Trujillo, A. Card. L. (1997, February 12). *VADEMECUM FOR CONFESSORS CONCERNING SOME ASPECTS OF THE MORALITY OF CONJUGAL LIFE.* Vademecum for confessors concerning some aspects of the morality of the conjugal life. https://www.vatican.va/roman_curia/pontifical_councils/family/documents/rc_pc_family_doc_12021997_vademecum_en.html

[23] Smoley, B. A., & Robinson, C. M. (2012). Natural family planning. *American family physician, 86*(10), 924–928.

[24] Center for Biologics Evaluation and Research. (2018, February 2). *Anthrax.* U.S. Food and Drug Administration. https://www.fda.gov/vaccines-blood-biologics/vaccines/anthrax#:~:text=The%20mortality%20rates%20from%20anthrax,that%20is%2080%25%20or%20higher.

anthrax infection with 99% efficacy.[25] This new device is studied by researchers and medical professionals from various universities and hospitals around the world by giving participants the device and putting them into the anthrax filled room. All results from the various institutions are published in academic publications and although they are of a similar quality, the results vary greatly. Some studies show one out of every hundred people will be infected and some show one out of four.

You'll either be protected 99% or 75% of the time.

Here's the question: If I give you the new device, would you enter the anthrax room?

Personally, I'd laugh in the face of the researchers and run away. Replication of results is the hallmark of a reliable study. I repeat: if you want to show that a study can be trusted, replicate it. If everyone is getting different results, the data are unreliable.

(Which is also a great tip to debunk bad data in an argument.)

I used inhaled anthrax as an example because it has an 80% fatality rate. A similar percentage, 85% of women who have unprotected sex, even occasionally, will end up pregnant within a year.

Want to avoid this life altering event? NFP might protect you better than even the most effective birth control modern medicine has to offer. Or it might have a 25% chance of leaving you with a baby/lifelong responsibility.

Why the huge discrepancy? I can't tell you for sure, but I do know that NFP relies heavily on education, understanding, and adherence to

---

[25] The idea of a new respirator for anthrax is completely made up for this thought experiment. This is not a real thing and is not intended to mimic any real device.

detailed monitoring tasks. Apps can help reduce those problems by providing high quality education, reminders, and a reliable place to store data. The Natural Cycles app claims to increase NFP efficacy to 93% with typical use, but again, I had a hard time finding more than the original source (promoted by the producers of the app) replicating those results.

The intersection of abortion and natural family planning: Apps that allow users to track menstrual cycles for NFP or other purposes provide a digital log of when a women is most likely fertile and when she should be (or is) menstruating. If a person tracks her period reliably and then chooses to have an abortion, that abortion could be identified by altered or delayed cycle times in her preferred app. This specific topic went viral with the overturn of Roe v. Wade in 2022. As some states made abortion a criminal offense, people began to question what could be used as evidence to convict or imprison a woman who chooses abortion. Alternatively, in states that do not convict women, people who provide aid or advice related to a procedure may be jailed or heavily fined for their role in the act.

Some digital data that may incriminate a woman or abortion provider if a warrant was approved to search her digital devices:
- Receipts or proof of payment for the procedure including bank statements
- Email or calendar reminders of appointments
- Text and chat messages about the experience or pregnancy
- Period tracker data

Just like it would be incredibly difficult to argue for, or against, the protection device in the anthrax example, it would be hard to argue for, or against, NFP in any meaningful way. The truth is, until large scale studies with replicable, reliable results are available, neither side of this argument really has enough data to stand on.

That being said, NFP is a great way to *increase* your chances of conceiving if you're trying to get pregnant (rather than trying to avoid it). It's highly recommended for women who are considering fertility treatments and can be an excellent tool to try if you're not ready to pursue IVF.

Things that don't prevent pregnancy

While NFP might be a good backup option for some women, the majority of couples looking to prevent pregnancy using hormonal or barrier methods. If these tools start to become unavailable, women will still try to prevent pregnancy with traditional remedies. Unfortunately, most of the folk remedies out there are only as effective as a hope and a wish at the end of the day.

Jumping after sex - While it might be great exercise, jumping up and down will not shake sperm out of a vagina. The fluid sperm floats in will typically exit the vaginal canal sometime after sex and people may see drips coming down their legs if they pop up and start jumping around after the act. However, this fluid does not carry all the sperm with it. Remember, those squirmy suckers can grab on to the uterine wall or scurry up into the cervix faster than you can stand up and start hopping around. No reliable method for removing sperm from the vagina or cervical canal has ever been discovered.

Douching after sex - Douching is generally not recommended by gynecologists. It can upset the balance of bacteria in the vaginal tract and only reaches the vagina, not the cervix or uterus, where sperm is headed.

Black Cohosh - Found in most health food stores, this herb is commonly used to help with irregular periods and symptoms of menopause with a fair amount of reliability.[26] That being said, I could not find any human data that proves cause and effect between this herb and contraceptive or abortifacient outcomes.

Cotton Root Bark - The Encyclopedia of Toxicity discusses the primary compound, Gossypol, in cotton root related to its use in female and male reproduction.[27] In China, it was once widely used by men to

---

[26] U.S. Department of Health and Human Services. (2020, June 3). *Office of dietary supplements - black cohosh*. NIH Office of Dietary Supplements. https://ods.od.nih.gov/factsheets/BlackCohosh-HealthProfessional/

[27] Wexler, P. (Ed.). (2014). *Encyclopedia of Toxicology. ScienceDirect* (3rd ed.). Elsevier Academic Press. Retrieved July 6, 2023, from

decrease fertility and while it was assumed to be effective, negative side effects including nutritional deficiency caused it to fall out of favor. In women, it's been known to help with menopause, endometriosis and myomas. However, finding any data about its use as a female contraceptive or abortifacient was difficult.

Pennyroyal -

"Sit and drink Pennyroyal Tea
Distill the life that's inside of me
Sit and drink Pennyroyal Tea
I'm anemic royalty
Give me a Leonard Cohen afterworld
So I can sigh eternally"

- Kurt Cobain, Pennyroyal Tea

Do not, I repeat, **do not** consume pennyroyal post-sex as a contraceptive or post-conception as an abortifacient. Yes, it *may* terminate a pregnancy, but only because it contains a highly toxic compound, pulegone[28] (banned by the FDA as a food additive, but still found in e-cigarettes and some menthol tobacco) that will poison you. As your organs shut down, and your heart/lungs stop working, and your liver gives up, an embryo is likely to be harmed and aborted in the process. This works much the same as any other poisoning; pregnancies can be collateral damage when maternal health and/or life is severely threatened. If you're someone who uses pennyroyal in essential oils, do not consume those oils. Do not make tea out of this. Do not eat it. Just don't put it inside your body at all, for any reason.

---

https://www.sciencedirect.com/referencework/9780123864550/encyclopedia-of-toxicology.

[28] Caputo, L., Cornara, L., Raimondo, F. M., De Feo, V., Vanin, S., Denaro, M., Trombetta, D., & Smeriglio, A. (2021). *Mentha pulegium* L.: A Plant Underestimated for Its Toxicity to Be Recovered from the Perspective of the Circular Economy. *Molecules (Basel, Switzerland)*, *26*(8), 2154. https://doi.org/10.3390/molecules26082154

If these remedies don't work, what should someone do if their birth control method fails? This is where emergency contraceptives come in.

Chapter 5

Emergency Contraception

"Contraception stops a woman from becoming pregnant. The Plan B pill kills a baby in the womb once a woman is already pregnant."
- Marjorie Taylor Greene, US House of Representatives[29]

Nope. That's not how that works.

Plan B, also known as levonorgestrel or the morning-after pill, is usually brought up in the same discussion as abortion but if you noticed, we're not in the abortion chapter of this book. Why? Because this medication is not an abortifacient.

---

[29] Campoamor, D. (2021, June 25). *Marjorie Taylor Greene is as wrong about plan B as she is about everything else*. Does Marjorie Taylor Greene Know What Plan B Is? https://www.refinery29.com/en-us/2021/06/10546850/marjorie-taylor-greene-plan-b-abortion-pill-difference

I repeat. This medication has nothing to do with abortion. In fact, its only real use is preventing an egg from entering the fallopian tubes in the first place, which is why the same exact compound (levonorgestrel) is used in a once-a-day oral contraceptive pill under the brand name Seasonale.

Even by the widest stretch of a "personhood" definition, an unfertilized oocyte sitting in a person's ovaries is not considered a distinct human. Something like 35 oocytes will die every day, and nearly 1000 oocytes will perish in a month due to natural processes alone (If you need a reminder, flip back to the ovulatory cycle and read the part regarding oocyte maturation).[30] Most eggs never even glimpse a chance of fertilization.

Now that we got that out of the way, imagine this: It's your anniversary and after a beautiful dinner, you and your partner decide to have consensual adult 'bonding' time.[31] After many years, you continue to use condoms as a primary form of birth control since they're easier to remember than a pill. This particular night when the deed is done, the condom slides off, depositing all those unwanted sperm into the vaginal canal. Try as hard as you may, there's no catching those super-fast swimmers once they've been released – one study found sperm in the fallopian tubes just 5 minutes after insemination![32] Those little swimmers are the Michael Phelps of biology. And they're persistent too, most sources say they can survive 3-5 days in a woman's reproductive tract and still fertilize an egg.

Think this is an unlikely scenario? Well, in addition to being a true story from my own life, the stats for condom "slippage" come in at around

---

[30] Silber, S. J. (2022, January 7). *Beating your biological clock - understanding female eggs*. The Infertility Center of St. Louis. https://www.infertile.com/infertility-101/female-infertility/beating-biological/

[31] Sex. I'm talking about sex.

[32] Ahlgren, M. (2010). Sperm Transport to and Survival in the Human Fallopian Tube. Gynecologic and Obstetric Investigation, 6(3-4), 206-214.

2.0%-2.7% of condom users.[33] That means 27 people out of 1,000 will have a condom fall off. If you refer back to the efficacy of birth control methods in the last chapter, you'll notice that the real world fail rate of condoms is *eighteen* percent. 18 out of 100 women using condoms in a year will end up pregnant.

When mistakes happen. Levonorgestrel is a good backup.

So, what is it? While there are two forms of emergency contraceptive pills approved by the FDA, we'll cover Plan B first as it's the most recognizable brand name in the United States. This pill is similar to daily birth control pills, but it acts on a much more immediate basis.

We already covered how progestins (the main ingredient in monthly birth control pills) are progesterone analogs. Levonorgestrel, another chemical lookalike in the progestogen family, binds to Pgr receptors, tricking the body into thinking there's more progesterone being produced than there actually is.

By taking a single 1.5 milligram pill of levonorgestrel, progesterone receptors are flooded with this imitator, and the same process is triggered as would be if natural ovulation just occurred. The body assumes an egg has been released, so it refrains from releasing another. The developing follicle(s) in the ovary will fail to complete maturation and won't pop out of their Graafian follicles, instead disintegrating over time. Because an egg is not released, any sperm that made it into the reproductive tract will eventually give up and die off, leaving the woman pregnancy-free.

The main mechanism of action here is to *prevent* ovulation. But what happens if ovulation has already occurred and that Graafian follicle just

---

[33] Grady, W. R., & Tanfer, K. (1994). Condom breakage and slippage among men in the United States. *Family planning perspectives*, *26*(3), 107–112.

popped out an oocyte that's now being brushed along the fallopian tubes to meet the flood of incoming sperm?

What now?

Well, you're probably out of luck. Some researchers have argued there *may* be post-fertilization effects of levonorgestrel, but that's been pretty well disproven. Repeatedly (remember replication = reliability). ACOG wrote in their official statement, "...the levonorgestrel-only regimen have been shown to inhibit or delay ovulation ...review of the evidence suggests that emergency contraception is unlikely to prevent implantation of a fertilized egg."[34] Additionally, there are two separate studies (both small scale, one with 99[35] and another with 148 participants[36]) that show nearly identical results when testing the efficacy of this medication when taken before and after ovulation. Both studies determined the day of ovulation for participants and tracked when in her cycle a woman had unprotected sex. Next, they used statistical data to determine how many women would become pregnant *without* intervention under similar circumstances. Then, they compared the number of pregnancies that actually happened after taking emergency contraceptive pills with the number of pregnancies that would be expected without intervention.

---

[34] Emergency contraception. Practice Bulletin No. 152. American College of Obstetricians and Gynecologists. Obstet Gynecol 2015;126:e1–11.
[35] Novikova, N., Weisberg, E., Stanczyk, F. Z., Croxatto, H. B., & Fraser, I. S. (2007). Effectiveness of levonorgestrel emergency contraception given before or after ovulation--a pilot study. *Contraception*, *75*(2), 112–118. https://doi.org/10.1016/j.contraception.2006.08.015
[36] Noé, G., Croxatto, H. B., Salvatierra, A. M., Reyes, V., Villarroel, C., Muñoz, C., Morales, G., & Retamales, A. (2011). Contraceptive efficacy of emergency contraception with levonorgestrel given before or after ovulation. *Contraception*, *84*(5), 486–492. https://doi.org/10.1016/j.contraception.2011.03.006

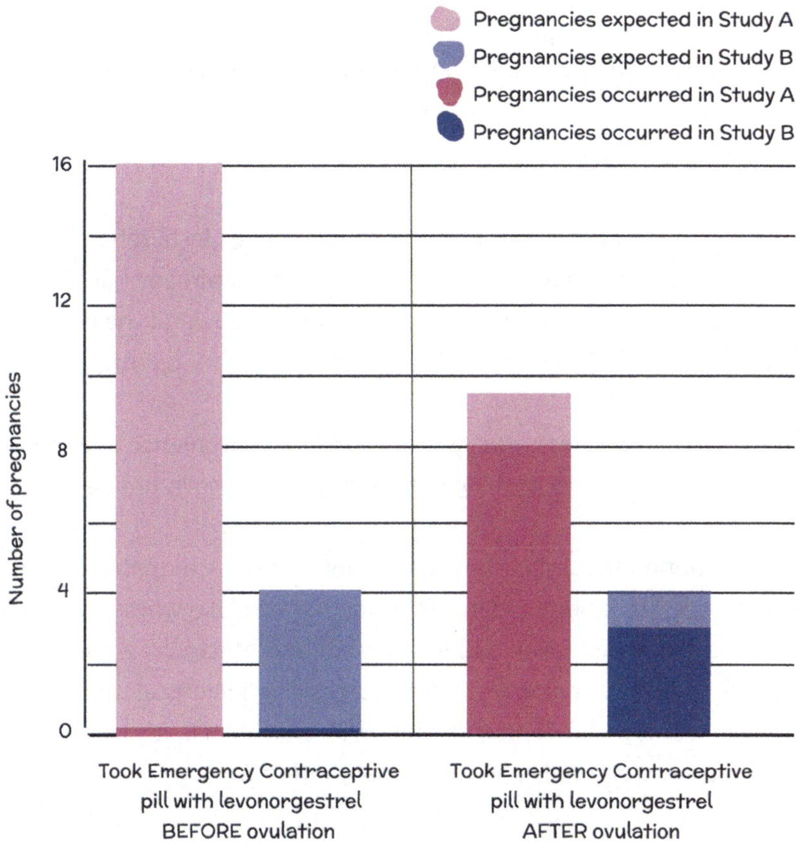

In the first study, the group of 34 women who had not yet ovulated but had unprotected sex during the fertile period of their cycle (right before ovulation) would be expected to have four pregnancies without intervention. However, after taking an emergency contraceptive pill including levonorgestrel, none occurred. In the second study, a group of 103 women did the same and although 16 pregnancies would be expected, none occurred. Based on this, Plan B/levonorgestrel seems to be highly effective.

Now look at the numbers for those who took the same dosage *after* ovulation, 8.7 pregnancies would be expected in one study and 4 in the other. How many occurred? 8 and 3. Levonorgestrel did pretty much nothing to prevent pregnancy in the group who had unprotected sex and then took Levonorgestrel *after* ovulation. This not only demonstrates [the likelihood of] high efficacy if taken before the LH surge/ovulation, but also the likelihood that levonorgestrel does a whole lot of nadda after ovulation.[37]

In our slippage example, the egg is hurtling towards fertilization and Plan B isn't able to do much about that if ovulation already happened. The ability to prevent pregnancy vs. not could be down to the hour of condom failure or the time of day a clinic or pharmacy opens.

What other accident can change from a mild inconvenience to a lifetime of responsibility due to nothing but a slight difference in timing?

A second option that might be slightly more effective in that situation is ulipristal acetate (abbreviation: UA, trade name: ELLA) which is thought to be effective when taken within 5 days of unprotected sex, even if ovulation has occurred. While most sources claim ulipristal acetate primarily works by preventing ovulation just like Plan B, it's important to note that it's structurally and functionally different.

First, ulipristal is not a progesterone analog. It's a progesterone receptor modulator. On a biochemical level, it binds to Pgr receptors so progesterone cannot, blocking the normal effect of progesterone. It turns out, ovulation can be prevented by adding progestins to the system with levonorgestrel *or* removing the effect of progesterone with UA.

What?

---

[37]Remember, small scale studies always need to be taken with a grain of salt. The fact the first study could be replicated by a different team with a different patient set is promising since replication is key. However, the results would be stronger if we had a larger pool of data. Always think about your sources!

This is where it's important to note that it's not just an increase or decrease in hormones that cause the ovulatory cycle to progress, it's the *correct* amount of hormones that are needed.

The other thing to know about ulipristal is that pre-ovulatory action alone doesn't account for UA's high efficacy. One study shows that when taken within 36 hours of ovulation, only 8% of women experienced an anti-ovulatory effect (before that time period, it strongly inhibits ovulation just like levonorgestrel).[38] This means that an oocyte is still popping out of the Graafian follicle to live its days out as an egg floating down the female reproductive tract. However, the same study states that Ella remains about 80% effective despite the fact that it does not prevent ovulation.[39]

Fair evaluation of facts: For the sake of accuracy, I want to acknowledge that ulipristal acetate *may* have abortifacient properties (yet unknown).
- A Phase 4 Clinical Trial was approved in Egypt to test the "Use of Ulipristal Acetate in Induction of Second Trimester Missed Abortion". As of writing, results have not been posted.
- A current study is recruiting volunteers in Mexico for "Evaluating ulipristal acetate and misoprostol for induced abortion through 63 days of pregnancy"
- Mifepristone is also a progesterone receptor modulator and is used in medical abortions. Not all medications in the same class have identical effects, but they are often comparable.
- Ulipristal and mifepristone were equally likely to induce abortion in guinea pigs. *Remember, although a promising starting point, animal studies often do not translate to human effects.*

1. Evaluating ulipristal acetate and misoprostol for induced abortion through 63 days of pregnancy. ISRCTNregistry. (2022, September 2). https://www.isrctn.com/ISRCTN35625202
2. Use of Ulipristal Acetate in Induction of Second Trimester Missed Abortion. ClinicalTrials.gov. (2021, August 4). https://clinicaltrials.gov/-study/NCT04989400
3. European Medicines Agency. (2009). (rep.). CHMP ASSESSMENT REPORT FOR EllaOne. Retrieved July 6, 2023, from https://www.ema.eu-ropa.eu/en/documents/assessment-report/ella-one-epar-public-assessment-report_en.pdf.

How can that be?
Some researchers believe that ulipristal acetate prevents the

---

[38] Mozzanega, B., & Nardelli, G. B. (2019). UPA and LNG in emergency contraception: the information by EMA and the scientific evidences indicate a prevalent anti-implantation effect. *The European journal of contraception & reproductive health care : the official journal of the European Society of Contraception*, *24*(1), 4–10. https://doi.org/10.1080/13625187.2018.1555662
[39] After reading the study, I'm not 100% sure where the 80% effective figure comes from but it's repeated in many sources. So keep in mind the 80% number is not backed up with a primary source.

endometrial lining from producing its final embryo-friendly layers[40] or possibly stalls production of proteins needed for successful growth of an embryo. At the end of the day, there's no final consensus on what the additional mechanisms of action are for medications like Ella. And as much as there's a need for additional emergency contraceptives, it would be inappropriate to not mention that there are currently multiple studies recruiting volunteers to test if ulipristal acetate would be useful if given in tandem with other medications that induce abortions and/or induce labor in pregnancy.

Despite being lumped in with Plan B, which works pre-ovulation and has no abortifacient properties, it's important to acknowledge that we can't definitively say the same for ulipristal acetate. Although it would be medically inaccurate to say this medication *does* have abortifacient or post-ovulatory effects, we also cannot confirm it does not. The truth is, we don't really know for sure.

Let's take a break to discuss just how little we know about how so many medications work. At the end of the day, pharmaceutical developers are just throwing theories at problems and seeing what sticks. Those theories are extremely well-developed and backed by decades, or even centuries, of science but because the body is an infinitely complex structure, no one ever really knows what is going to happen when we introduce a new chemical into the system. Instead, drug developers take all the knowledge they have (altering progesterone levels can prevent ovulation) and apply it when developing a medication (let's block progesterone receptors). Then they see if it works. First, it's tested in a lab, then maybe on animals, then if everything is promising, we slowly start testing it at low doses in humans. It takes years to narrow down if a

---

[40]Lira-Albarrán, S., Durand, M., Barrera, D., Vega, C., Becerra, R. G., Díaz, L., García-Quiroz, J., Rangel, C., & Larrea, F. (2018). A single preovulatory administration of ulipristal acetate affects the decidualization process of the human endometrium during the receptive period of the menstrual cycle. *Molecular and cellular endocrinology*, *476*, 70–78. https://doi.org/10.1016/j.mce.2018.04.010

medication will work and even after that, when it's introduced on a wide scale, side effects might pop up that were never encountered during testing.

For example, Thalidomide was once used for nausea in pregnancy with great success. In short, it had its desired effect. Unfortunately, the medical community discovered only too late that it also caused severe birth defects by degrading a bunch of proteins that help activate and deactivate genes. This was causing a gene that stimulates the development of limbs to be turned off, causing missing or deformed body parts in newborn babies.[41] The drug had its intended effect but still caused issues by also binding to unexpected proteins.

In the case of UA, it's preventing pregnancy pre-ovulation as planned. However, we're still determining if there are other effects and what they are (potentially, changes in the endometrium post-ovulation).

I mention this because the moral line for some people that divides OK and not OK may be drawn between pre-ovulatory and post-ovulatory effects. I want to make sure that line is clearly marked for ethical clarity

Emergency contraceptive option #2: The IUD
Also known as a type of long-acting reversible contraception.

How about stuffing some silkworm guts up into a person's uterus to prevent pregnancy? Thankfully we've come a long way since the first version of an intrauterine device (IUD), but the history of its development is written in surprising detail – including old timey medical drawings! – in Smithsonian Magazine.[42]

---

[41] Katherine A Donovan, Jian An, Radosław P Nowak, Jingting C Yuan, Emma C Fink, Bethany C Berry, Benjamin L Ebert, Eric S Fischer (2018) Thalidomide promotes degradation of SALL4, a transcription factor implicated in Duane Radial Ray syndrome eLife 7:e38430 https://doi.org/10.7554/eLife.38430
[42] Copeland, L. (2017, June 15). *From medical pariah to feminist icon: The story of the IUD*. Smithsonian.com.

Nowadays we have copper and hormonal IUDs, which are categorized as both a long-term form of reliable birth control and a type of emergency contraception if placed shortly after unprotected sex. Aside from abstinence and an implant, the IUD is the most reliable form of contraceptive with a real-world efficacy of 99%.

Why doesn't every womb that's not eagerly awaiting a baby have one of these installed? As an emergency contraceptive, an IUD can be inserted up to 5 days after unprotected sex. However, the average wait time for an OBGYN appointment was found to be 31.4 days in 2022.[43] While that's fine for non-emergency use, it's not helpful for those in a time crunch. Unlike Plan B which can be purchased at any pharmacy (at the time of writing this book), inserting an IUD is a proper medical

> Despite the fact that Planned Parenthood logged 2,193,205 appointments related to "birth control information and services," funding for their clinics remains a politically charges topic.
> **Example:** Title X is a grant that was established in 1970 to provide access to family planning and reproductive health services. It has never covered abortion. What it does cover is cervical and breast cancer screenings, birth control, contraceptive education, wellness exams, STI and HIV testing. 41% of Title X patients are treated through Planned Parenthood. Yet the debate over these funds continues.
>
> **2019** - Title X facilities were banned from discussing abortion as an option to any patient. No referrals allowed. In response, Planned Parenthood had to turn down funding as providers were unable to openly discuss all reproductive options with patients who asked and tranfer patients outside of Title X visits when needed.
>
> **2021** - The "gag order" was reversed. Title X money still does NOT cover abortion, but providers are once again allowed to answer questions openly and refer patients to an abortion provider (outside of Title X funding) when requested.

---

https://www.smithsonianmag.com/science-nature/medical-pariah-feminist-icon-story-iud-180963699/

[43]Baicker K, Chandra A. Medicare spending, the physician workforce, and beneficiaries' quality of care. *Health Aff (Millwood)*. 2004;23(suppl W4):184-197.

procedure. An alternative to scheduling with a standard OBGYN is to visit a clinic like Planned Parenthood that allows walk-ins and appointments on short notice. [44]

Once a person gets an appointment, they can choose either a hormonal or copper device. Both types are small T-shaped objects that are inserted into the uterus, but the hormonal options also release progestin for up to 7 years as added protection.

Does it hurt?

I once heard the pain of insertion described by a dear friend as "worse than labor contractions, but much shorter and definitely worth it." Most physicians still claim the insertion of an IUD is only accompanied by "some discomfort", which is true for the majority of women, but studies have shown that 11%-17% of women experience "substantial" pain. I bring this up specifically because women are shown over and over to receive less pain medication than men in pain-equivalent procedures.

Despite that, standard pain control offerings include nothing more than intracervical numbing gel, a paracervical block (injections of lidocaine on and surrounding the cervix), ibuprofen/advil, and/or tramadol (a light opiate). In review of available literature, it turned out that all of the listed pain management options were no more helpful than placebos.[45]
If a patient specifically requests conscious sedation or IV sedation, a provider may agree but this is not yet common practice.
The only positive here is that NSAIDS (like Aleve) may offer slight pain relief after the procedure.

---

[44] Parenthood, P. (n.d.). *Title X: Affordable birth control and reproductive health care*. Planned Parenthood Action Fund. https://www.plannedparenthoodaction.org/issues/health-care-equity/title-x#:~:text=Federal%20Title%20X%20funding%20was,basic%2C%20preventive%20reproductive%20health%20care.

[45] Gemzell-Danielsson, K., Mansour, D., Fiala, C., Kaunitz, A. M., & Bahamondes, L. (2013). Management of pain associated with the insertion of intrauterine contraceptives. *Human reproduction update*, *19*(4), 419–427. https://doi.org/10.1093/humupd/dmt022

I don't want to scare anyone seeking an IUD, but I *do* want anyone reading this, or the partners of readers, to feel empowered to discuss IV sedation with your doctor if you feel it's the right choice for you. Your insurance may even cover it. And if not, maybe it's time to start asking why it doesn't.

How does insertion happen?

To insert an IUD, a medical provider will use a speculum to open the vaginal canal (remember, the vagina is like a collapsed tube of toothpaste with the sides touching one another when not in use) and use a long thin measuring device to determine the length of the uterus looking for an ideal depth of 6-9cm. Below this range, the risk of IUD expulsion increases and there's nothing worse than having an IUD dislodge after going through the inconvenience and pain of having one placed.

After taking measurements, a medical provider will load the insertion device by folding the arms of the T-shaped IUD downward and sliding it into the tube-like insertion device. The entire tube then goes up through the vaginal canal, into the cervix, and up to the very top of the uterus. Once there, the bottom of the insertion tube is pushed upwards, causing the IUD to slide out of the top of the tube until the T arms spring open in place. Then the insertion tube is removed and the IUD is left inside with two strings dangling through the cervical os. These strings provide a reliable way for women and physicians to ensure proper placement of the IUD in the future. It's a similar mechanism to the insertion of a tampon just much further up the reproductive tract.

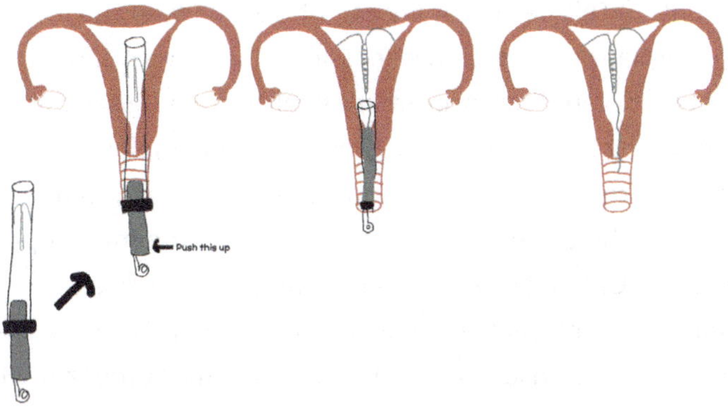

How does it work?

For copper IUDs, once it's in place, a small amount of copper ions constantly leak into the reproductive tract. These ions are like kryptonite to sperm, rendering them more or less immobile so they cannot swim to their intended target.[46] The presence of a foreign object can also cause a local inflammatory response which makes the uterus less hospitable to implantation.

For hormonal IUDs like Mirena (brand name sold in the United States), about 20 micrograms of levonorgestrel will be released each day[47] which acts just as it would in any other form of birth control by thickening the cervical mucus and suppressing ovulation. These plastic devices also cause an inflammatory response that may make the uterus inhospitable to fertilized eggs.

That's cool, but when would I ever need to argue about IUDs?

In 2014, a congressional candidate, Bob Beauprez, said that IUDs were

---

[46] Chattopadhyay, P., Magdanz, V., Hernández-Meliá, M., Borchert, K.B.L., Schwarz, D. and Simmchen, J. (2022), Size-Dependent Inhibition of Sperm Motility by Copper Particles as a Path toward Male Contraception. Adv. NanoBiomed Res., 2: 2100152. https://doi.org/10.1002/anbr.202100152

[47] Bayer Healthcare Pharmaceuticals. Mirena [package insert]. U.S. Food and Drug Administration website. https://www.accessdata.fda.gov/drugsatfda_docs/label/2008/021225s019lbl.pdf. Published 2018. Accessed 22/6/2023.

abortifacients.[48] This particular argument was made in the context of abortion, but has popped up in discussions about what should and should not be covered by government healthcare programs since. While this *is* a tempting talking point, IUDs only prevent implantation of a fertilized egg into the uterus. They do not kill an embryo that has implanted into the uterine wall. In fact, Paragard, the main copper IUD provider in the United States specifically lists pregnancy as a contraindication for insertion, meaning no one with an active pregnancy would be eligible for insertion. If a woman becomes pregnant while using an IUD, it should be removed by a physician according to the provider's guidelines.

The remaining argument is that if sperm has already reached an egg and that egg is fertilized immediately before IUD placement, the IUD may create a hostile uterine environment due to the inflammatory response in the uterus. That fertilized egg will then perish and be expelled during the next menstrual cycle instead of implanting. While this *can* happen, it's really only relevant during the first month if inserted as an emergency contraceptive. Studies have shown that because copper ions are found throughout the human genital tract of IUD users, sperm is severely damaged when it enters the cervix and will never reach the egg in the first place. Additionally, some researchers have speculated that there are also negative effects on female oocytes once they've been released into the fallopian tubes (oocytes that remain inside the ovaries are not impacted). That means if a person with an IUD is having regular unprotected sex, you're unlikely to find fertilized eggs in their reproductive tracts regardless of how much sex they have.[49] Both the eggs and sperm are negatively affected so fertilization won't happen.

---

[48] Frank, J. (2016, June 10). *Bob Beauprez's IUD Remark in debate generates controversy*. The Denver Post. https://www.denverpost.com/2014/10/01/bob-beauprezs-iud-remark-in-debate-generates-controversy/

[49] Ortiz, M. E., Croxatto, H. B., & Bardin, C. W. (1996). Mechanisms of action of intrauterine devices. *Obstetrical & gynecological survey*, *51*(12 Suppl), S42–S51. https://doi.org/10.1097/00006254-199612000-00014

But what happens if a contraceptive device fails and a person finds themselves pregnant?

Chapter 6

What Really Happens at Six Weeks

It's time to take a break from contraception and think about conception. Before we get to the abortion chapter, we need to talk about something that makes even the most confident medical students cry in frustration: embryology. To determine if, and when, you have ethical issues with abortion, you really need to understand what's happening with the embryo. Not how big it is ("today your baby is the size of a cantaloupe!"), but what's *really* happening. Pretty much every politician or celebrity who has become a joke on social media in the pro-life/pro-choice debate has messed up this section.

Don't be a meme. Know your biology.

If we pick up where we left off in the previous chapter, sperm were deposited in the vagina and quickly swam up to the fallopian tubes looking for an egg to enter. About a day before that fateful event, an egg was released from the Graafian follicle in the ovaries, leaving behind a clump of cells called the corpus luteum. Now, that egg is being swept along the fallopian tubes when it meets some sperm. We'll skip all the science of fertilization and just get to the part where – BOOM – we have a zygote. One set of chromosomes from the egg and one from the sperm.

Did you know? One oddity about human oocytes that I feel a duty to point out in case anyone wants to assert their dominance over a high school biology teacher or come up with a great reproductive trivia question, is that even though we think of eggs and sperm as "haploid" (having only one set of chromosomes), eggs remain diploid (two sets of chromosomes) until fertilization. After a sperm enters the egg, it undergoes the final process of division (AKA meiosis II). This isn't super important for the subjects in this book, but most people think human eggs are haploid during their entire existence, and that's not true.

Once fertilization happens, a woman is already 2 weeks pregnant. "How is that?", you might ask. This is *very* important to understand when discussing cut-off dates for any type of post-fertilization procedure including abortion.Pregnancy is counted from the date of a woman's last period because we can usually narrow that down to a specific day, but we don't always know when fertilization happened. If a woman is entering her third week of pregnancy, she only has a "blastocyst" or a round clump of cells with a hollow, fluid-filled center, entering the uterus and getting ready to implant. It's not even nestled into her uterine lining yet.

When does it become a baby?

I think the real question here is, "When does life begin"? And for that, we have no easy answer. I do, however, find it useful to compare the beginning of life to the end of it. In the United States, 43 states have enacted the 1980 Determination of Death Act which defines the medical determination of death as, "an individual who has sustained either irreversible cessation of circulatory and respiratory functions or irreversible cessation of all functions of the entire brain, including the brainstem."

This means that if someone cannot breathe independently and does not have a heartbeat, they are dead. If someone has no brain function, they are dead. Both brain and cardio-respiratory failure equal medical death.

There's a growing number of physicians who argue this act should be amended because even when brainstem functions including the drive to breathe are gone in an unconscious person, the hypothalamus may still be releasing hormones to the pituitary.[50] You should remember this part of the brain from the ovulatory cycle; the hypothalamus releases GnRH to the pituitary which releases hormones like FSH and LH. Outside of reproduction, this hypothalamic-pituitary axis also releases additional hormones like growth hormone (GH), thyroid-stimulating hormone (TSH), prolactin, adrenocorticotropic hormone (ACTH), and vasopressin. The problem is that if "all functions of the entire brain" need to cease in order to declare death, a person may be entirely brain dead including all higher-level functions that comprise consciousness, but still have hormones released from the hypothalamus and pituitary glands. This small amount of functionality has nothing to do with life or breathing/circulation and does not impact the ability to survive but may preclude a physician from declaring death under the current act.

While looking at the next few pages, consider the definition of "life". Take into account the various developmental milestones and how difficult it is to determine when the heart is actually beating and when the brain is actually thinking.

Questions to ponder: If you believe life starts before the ability to independently breathe and pump blood throughout the body, does that make you reconsider the definition of "death" for older adults?

If you believe life does not begin until a baby is born, what medical facts would justify that argument?

Should "life" and "viability" (the ability of a fetus to survive outside the womb) be synonymous?

---

[50] Hannon, P. (2022, May 19). *Stanford biomedical ethicists among panelists updating law on definition of death*. Stanford Medicine News Center. https://med.stanford.edu/news/all-news/2022/05/definition-death-law.html

Now how about if someone is on a ventilator? How is death determined if they cannot independently breathe? For that, we have an apnea test. A person is first given 100% oxygen so their tissues and blood can be loaded with O_2. Then, they're removed from the ventilator. If they spontaneously breathe within 10 minutes, they're not dead. There's a great explanation of this process in the book, "Reaching Down the Rabbit Hole: A Renowned Neurologist Explains the Mystery and Drama of Brain Disease," by Dr. Allan H. Ropper and Brian David Burrell, that you can find excerpted on the Scientific America website if you want to know what it looks like in real life.[51]

Should we apply the same rules, the same apnea test, to an embryo or fetus? In which case, does life only occur after it can independently breathe, pump blood, and demonstrate at least basic brainstem activity? Keep this in mind as we explore what happens to the different organ systems as an embryo develops.

Development of an Embryo

Let's look at how an embryo comes to be a baby. Using a chronological chart, you can see the important milestones for development and how those milestones line up with common abortion cutoffs.

First, we have the journey from egg → zygote (a single cell, fertilized egg) → (a 16-cell clump) → blastula (a hollow ball of cells). Be sure to note the time after fertilization vs. the number of weeks pregnant as well as the location of events on the left side.

---

[51] Ropper, A., & Burrell, B. D. (2015). *Reaching down the Rabbit Hole: A renowned neurologist explains the mystery and drama of ... brain disease.* Griffin.

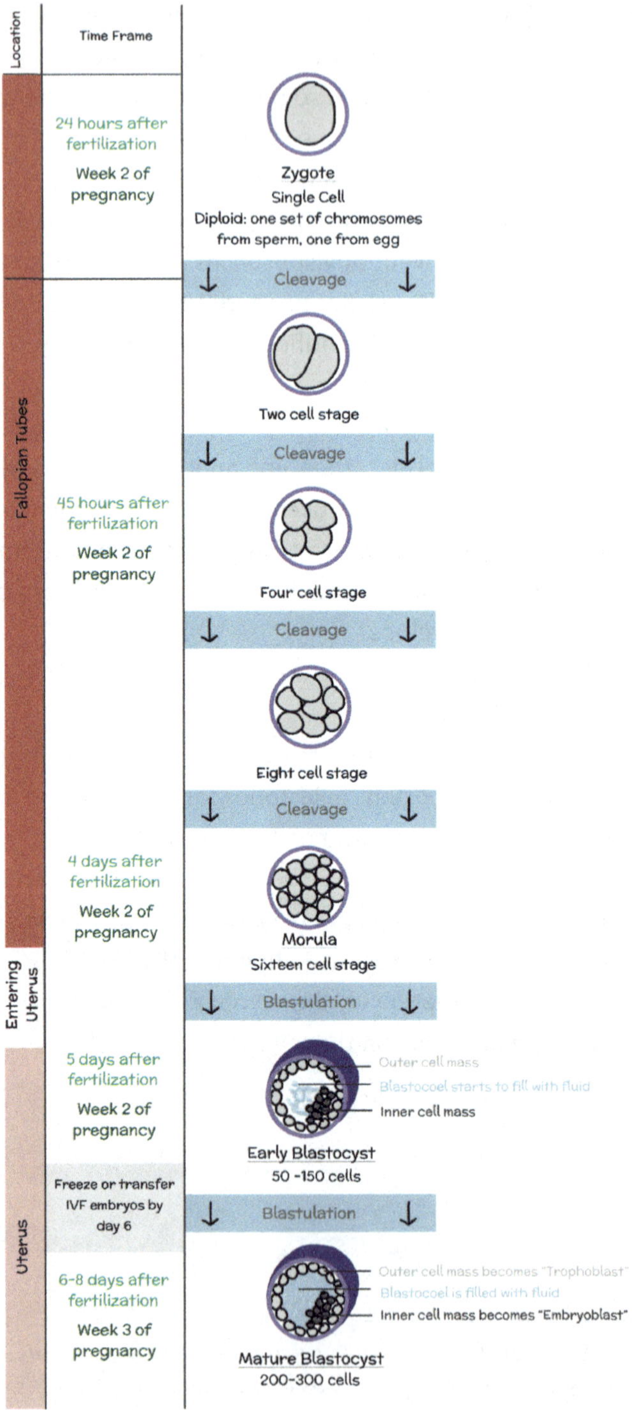

Location
Time Frame
Fallopian Tubes
24 hours after fertilization
Week 2 of pregnancy
Zygote
Single Cell
Diploid: one set of chromosomes from sperm, one from egg
Cleavage
Two cell stage
Cleavage
45 hours after fertilization
Week 2 of pregnancy
Four cell stage
Cleavage
Eight cell stage
Cleavage
4 days after fertilization
Week 2 of pregnancy
Morula
Sixteen cell stage
Entering Uterus
Blastulation
Uterus
5 days after fertilization
Week 2 of pregnancy
Outer cell mass
Blastocoel starts to fill with fluid
Inner cell mass
Early Blastocyst
50 -150 cells
Freeze or transfer IVF embryos by day 6
Blastulation
6-8 days after fertilization
Week 3 of pregnancy
Outer cell mass becomes "Trophoblast"
Blastocoel is filled with fluid
Inner cell mass becomes "Embryoblast"
Mature Blastocyst
200-300 cells

Implantation

Once a mature blastocyst exits the fallopian tubes and enters the uterus, it hatches (comes out of the zona pellucida) around day 6-7 after fertilization. On the egg's surface, selectins and pinopods stick out that allow the egg to attach to integrins and microvilli on the uterine cells. Think of these as hands sticking out of the egg, grabbing on to handles along the uterine wall. Once these grab each other, the egg starts invading the stratum functionalis of the uterus (which will now be called the **decidua**). Next, cells on the outside of the egg called "syncytiotrophoblasts" will expand into the uterine lining and start to break down, becoming an amorphous blob of cell guts. These cells release hCG which is the hormone that causes a positive pregnancy test (and, for the unfortunate ones, morning sickness). Remember this step, because if these cells grow out of control in a type of pregnancy called a "complete mole," and excessive hCG production will be one of the main signs.

To get nutrients to the embryo, coiled arteries in the uterine lining will grow towards the syncytiotrophoblast blob and start dripping blood into small puddles nearby. Eventually, these puddles become bigger, creating blood lakes called lacunae.

At the center of the syncytiotrophoblast blob, 'cytotrophoblast cells' line the growing cell mass. As time passes, the cytotrophoblast will grow outwards towards the maternal blood supply. In partial molar pregnancies these are the cells that grow out of control.

An extraembryonic mesoderm layer forms about 12 days after fertilization and this will eventually become the umbilical cord. Finally, a bilaminar (two-layered) disc is created with two sacs of fluid: the amniotic and yolk sacs. By day 14 after fertilization, week 4 of pregnancy, the embryo has implanted.

A placenta will eventually form around the end of the first trimester, at which point the corpus luteum will no longer be needed for hormone production.

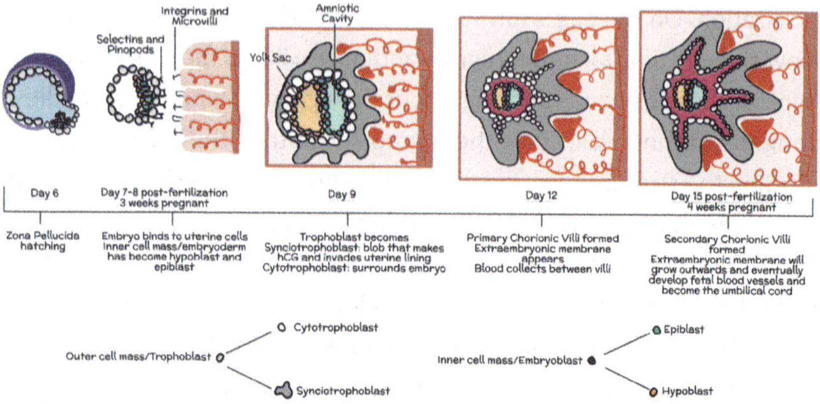

Implantation is usually the line people draw between "preventing pregnancy" and "ending pregnancy". Preventing an egg from being fertilized is considered contraception, but removing an embryo from the uterine lining may be considered abortion.

The gray area comes in when we prevent implantation. If a medication alters the uterine lining to prevent implantation of a fertilized embryo, are we preventing pregnancy or ending it?

Ways implantation can go wrong

If implantation happens with too much gusto, placental cells may grow into the deeper layers of the endometrium. In a healthy implantation, only the decidua should be invaded. If the placenta grows into the stratum basalis (bottom layer of uterine lining), we call it placenta accreta. If it gets to the myometrium (the muscular layer around the whole uterus), it's called placenta increta. And if a person is unlucky enough to have the placenta grow through the myometrium, it's placenta percreta. The deeper the placenta grows, the more complications it presents. In minor cases of placenta accreta, it's important to have extra blood on hand during labor and delivery to make sure excessive blood loss doesn't harm the mother. In cases of placenta increta or percreta, bleeding may be present later in pregnancy and in worst-case-scenarios, a hysterectomy might be needed after delivery if the uterus is too damaged when the placenta is removed.

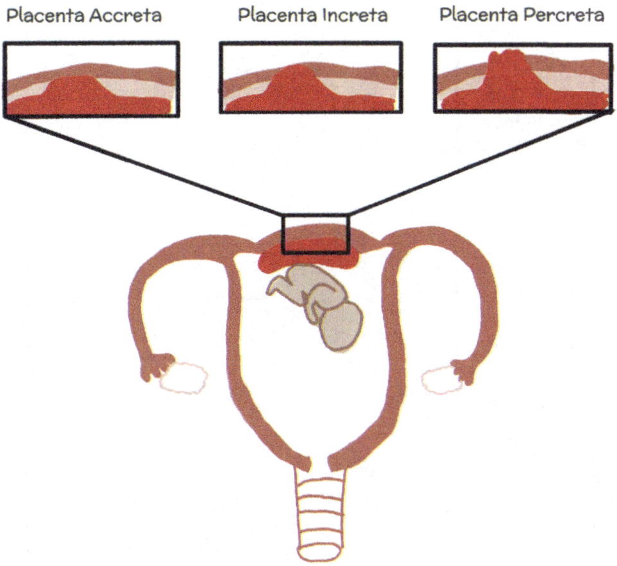

Alternatively, the placenta may grow to the right depth, but in the wrong place. If the fertilized egg attaches too low in the uterus and the placenta grows over the cervical opening, we have placenta previa. A pregnancy with a low-lying placenta will typically grow and develop normally but when it's time to deliver, a woman will have to give birth via c-section due to the fact the placenta is blocking the baby's exit route. If a woman does not receive prenatal care and placenta previa is not diagnosed before delivery, an attempt at vaginal delivery can be extremely dangerous and will not be successful. Surgery is the only reasonable solution.

Embryonic development

From here, let's follow the development of the embryo after implantation and through gastrulation. This process starts with a bilaminar disc containing an epiblast and hypoblast all the way through the development of a trilaminar (three-layered) disc containing the ectoderm, mesoderm, and endoderm. This disc sets up the developmental foundation for future organs and all cell differentiation.

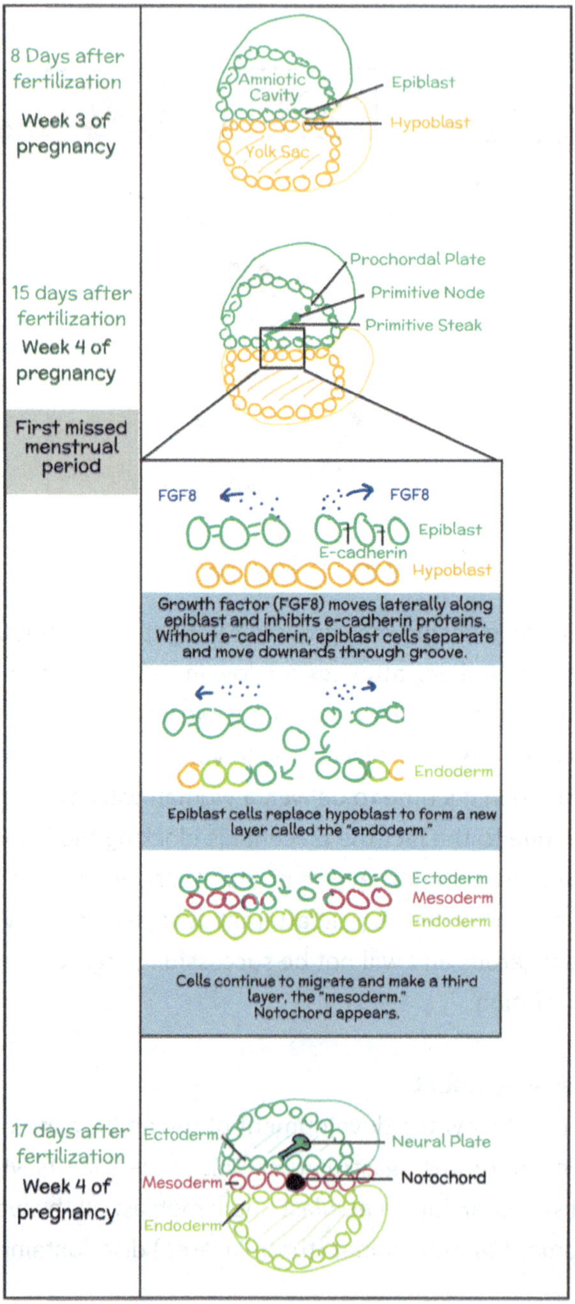

Note that it's not until Week 4 of pregnancy (14+ days after fertilization) that a person would miss a menstrual period. Given normal variances in menstruation, it's not until a few days, or even weeks, later that most people would take a pregnancy test if they weren't expecting to get pregnant. At this point, the embryo has only just implanted and has not started developing any organ systems yet.

From here onwards, a million things are happening in the embryo all at once in different locations. To get a full-size newborn in 9 months, things have to move fast. This is probably the most complicated part of the abortion debate for a few reasons: 1. When "life" begins isn't really answered by the anatomy, and 2. We know so much about the development of an embryo now that the sheer amount of detail is deeply overwhelming.

The next chart shows the basic development of the heart tube and neural tube in the center, with more detailed views of those structures to the side. Despite trying to cover the most important bits, some things have still been left out for ease of understanding and space.

Stage	Time	Embryonic and Fetal Development from Week 3-24
Embryo Stage - Teratogens most harmful	Day 23/Week 3 after fertilization Week 5 of pregnancy 1 week after the first missed period	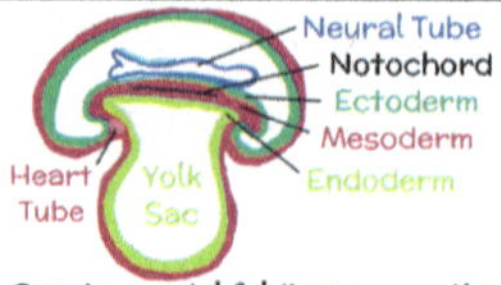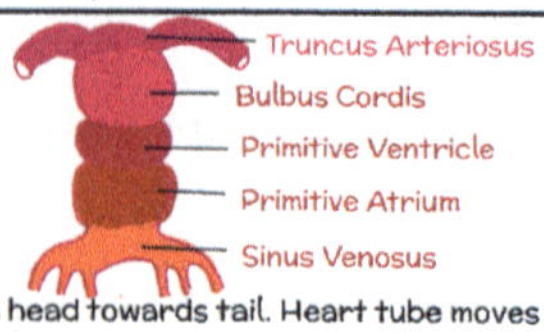 Cranio-caudal folding curves the embryo with head towards tail. Heart tube moves towards future thorax
	Week 4 after fertilization Week 6 of pregnancy	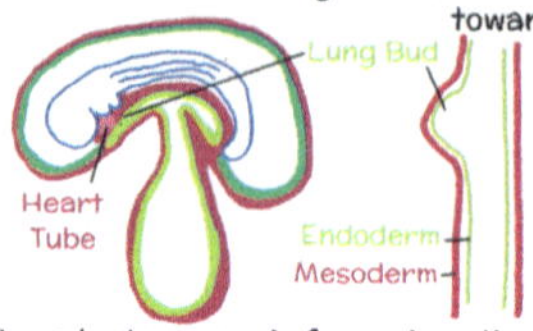 Lung bud appears in foregut portion of gut tube 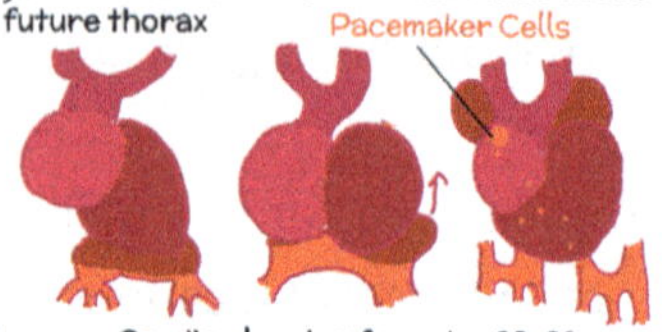 Cardiac looping from day 23-28: Primitive atria will move behind the primitive venticle and the upwards.
	Week 5 after fertilization Week 7 of pregnancy	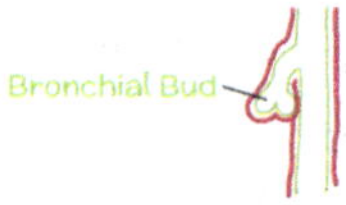 Lung bud becomes bronchial bud Trachioesophageal septum appears
	Week 6 after fertilization Week 8 of pregnancy	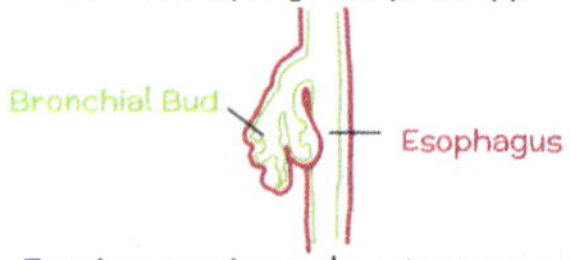 Tracheoesophageal septum separates bonchial bud from esophagus
	Week 8 after fertilization Week 10 of pregnancy	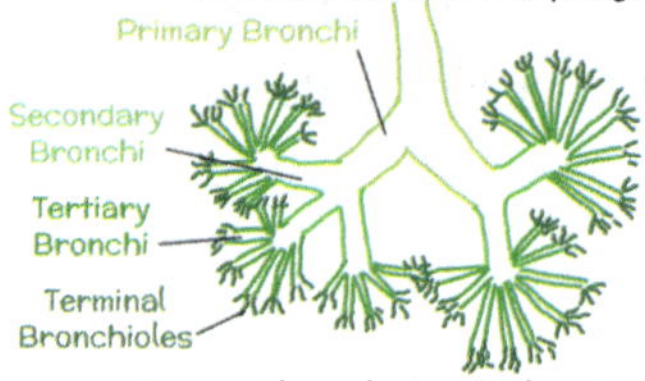 Pseudoglandular stage (week 6-16): Includes primary bronchi through terminal bronchioles 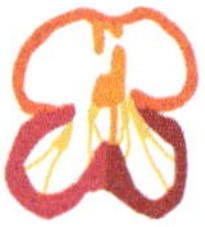 Atria and ventricle formed. SA node (pacemaker of adult heart) is identifiable. AV valves formed.
Fetal Stage	Week 16/Month 4 after fertilization Week 18/Month 4 of pregnancy	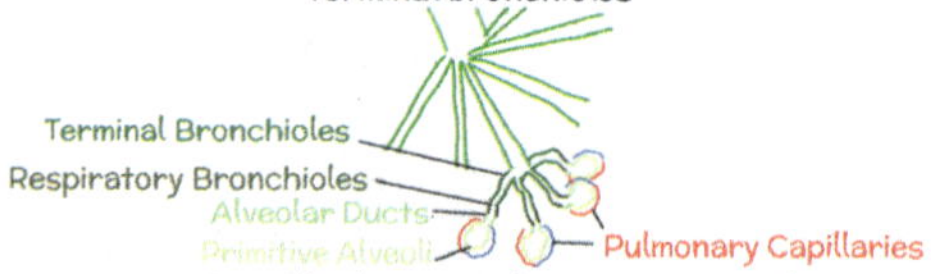 Cannalicular stage (week 16- week 26): Bronchi -> Primitive alveoli Primitive alveoli are made of cuboidal cells. Pulmonary cappillaries appear
	Week 24/Month 6 after fertilization Week 26/Month 6 of pregnancy	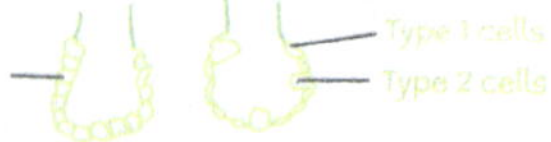 After week 26, cells lining aveoli become: Type 1 cells - flat, good for gas exchange Type 2 cells - produce surfactant

(week 5-26 of pregnancy)	Important Milestones

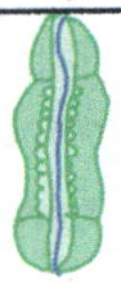

Neural tube closed by day 26

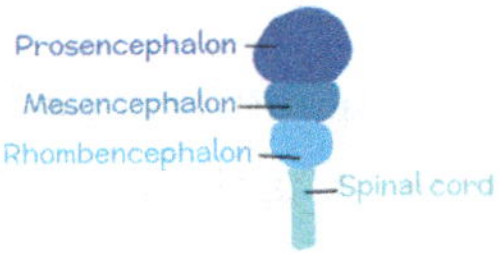

Primary Vesicle

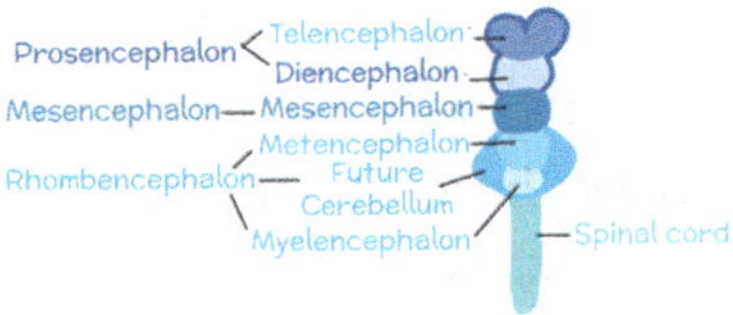

Secondary Vesicle

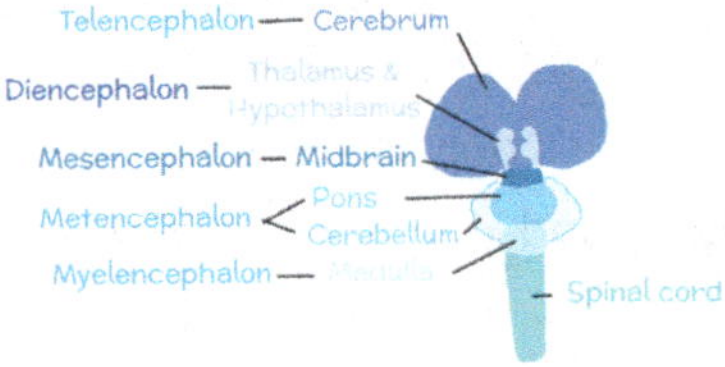

All parts of the brain are identifiable

First Trimester

Week 3 (week 5 of pregnancy):
Each system starts to develop:
The gut tube will become the esophagus, digestive system, lungs
The heart tube will become the heart
The neural tube will become the brain and nervous

Week 4 (week 6 of pregnancy):
Electrical activity identifiable in heart as pacemaker cells move from sinus arteriosis
Craniocaudal folding continues
Primary vesicle appears

Week 5 (week 7 of pregnancy):
Secondary vesicle forms
Bronchial bud starts developing

Week 6 (week 8 of pregnancy):
Electrical activity seen in secondary vesicle.
Movement may be seen on ultrasound

Week 8 (week 10 of pregnancy):
Heart looks like a heart with chambers and valves
After this week, the embryo is a fetus

Between weeks 8-12 (10-14 weeks of pregnancy): abnormalities may show up on ultrasound related to trisomies and neural tube defects

Second Trimester

Week 18 - 20 (16-18 weeks of pregnancy):
Maternal blood testg for neural tube defects and chromosomal abnormalities may be done

24 weeks/6 months:
Point of fetal viability
Fetal brain is functional but smooth, folding begins
Surfactant will start to be produced in lungs
Organs continue to develop and mature until birth

At about four weeks post-fertilization (6 weeks pregnant), all the tubes and buds needed for future organs will be developed. As you can see above, the heart tube is the first to develop and can actually start pumping blood before it becomes a mature heart.

The neural tube closes around day 26 after fertilization but is in no way a brain at this time. This tube will eventually become the nervous system, including the spinal cord.

The lungs are the last to develop and it's not until the fourth week that the gut tube and pharyngeal apparatus appear. The lungs and trachea will arise from the foregut of the gut tube, and the larynx (the general entry/exit point for food and air that includes your vocal cords and epiglottis) will come from the pharyngeal apparatus. The pharyngeal apparatus is a lumpy little thing towards the cranial/head end of the embryo that gives rise to pretty much everything in your face and neck that's not your brain: nerves, skin, glands, cartilage, muscle, etc.

From here, each tube is illustrated as if it's been pulled out of the embryo and layed out with the part closest to the head at the top. Imagine you're viewing these structures from above. Keep your eyes open for these highlights:

- Heart Highlights: Around day 22 post-fertilization (mid-week 5 of pregnancy), an electrical impulse referred to as a "heartbeat" may appear, but the organ it's being generated from doesn't really resemble a heart at all, it's more of a lumpy tube that's firing off some random electrical signals. At this stage, an embryo is not yet called a fetus, and it's only 2-3mm big. By 6 weeks, the heart loops around itself and kind of resembles something like a heart but inside the tube, there are still no separations between the chambers and there are no proper valves.
- Lung Highlights: Between week 5 and 6 of pregnancy, there are no lungs. Only lung buds. These are essentially still-useless

beginnings of lungs. Around 24/25 weeks of pregnancy, the lungs will be incredibly immature, but can sometimes result in a live birth with a surviving baby. Before that point, a baby cannot be born and breathe independently. One of the main factors for respiratory viability is the production of surfactant, which allows the alveoli to open without getting stuck together. The production of surfactant typically doesn't happen until after 24 weeks. If a person is expecting a premature birth, doctors may give corticosteroids to stimulate lung development in the baby and increase the likelihood they'll be able to breathe independently. Even after 24 weeks, premature babies often need some sort of mechanical ventilation to help move air into and out of their lungs.

- Brain Highlights: If we're looking at the brain, it's not until sometime between week 6-8 of pregnancy that some electrical activity might be observed in the beginning of the fetal brain. This allows an embryo to move. However, no structures for coordinated movement or thought will appear until the second trimester.

And here's where we should revisit the apnea test. One thing biology classes used to get wrong decades ago is teaching the respiratory system (lungs) and cardiovascular system (heart and blood vessels) as separate entities. Thankfully, my mom was a nursing instructor back in the day (100% NCLEX pass rates almost every year if anyone was wondering) and refused to teach anatomy and physiology in any way that wasn't integrated and function-first. From her, I learned that whenever someone mentions the respiratory system, they also meant the cardiovascular, and vice versa.

Here's the gist of adult cardio-respiratory function: We breathe air (with about 21% O_2 in it) through our mouth or nose, past our pharynx (the back of the throat), through the larynx, into the trachea (the tube that goes from the larynx to the lungs), and then through a bunch of narrowing tubes in the lungs until it reaches the alveoli. These tiny little sacs at the end of the passageway look like clusters of balloons on a microscopic scale. Because our alveoli have a slippery fluid called surfactant covering their inner walls, they can easily open to incoming air.

As air fills the alveoli, it diffuses across the very, very thin membrane into the surrounding capillaries (teeny tiny blood vessels). Carbon dioxide simultaneously exits from the capillaries into the alveoli and follows the same path in reverse and out through the mouth/nose.

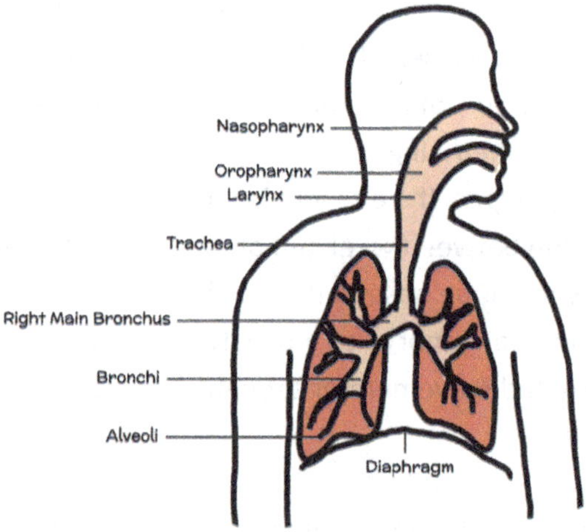

In the capillaries, oxygen is loaded onto a protein called hemoglobin, which relies on the help of iron to bind oxygen or carbon dioxide molecules. Each red blood cell (RBC) contains around 250-300 million hemoglobin proteins, so each RBC can carry a ton of oxygen and/or carbon dioxide. If a body cannot produce enough functional hemoglobin, as is the case if a person becomes iron deficient or has a dangerous genetic disorder called beta thalassemia, oxygen cannot be loaded onto red blood cells and carried around the body.

From the capillaries, red cells carrying their oxygen-laden hemoglobin will travel out of the lungs, through the short pulmonary veins, and into the heart. From here, the heart muscle does its job of pumping that oxygenated blood around the body to tissues, and less oxygenated blood from the tissues back to the lungs. The physical act of the heart pumping blood through its chambers and causing the valves of the heart to open and close is what makes a person's heartbeat. When you listen to someone's chest with a stethoscope this is what you're trying to hear – the valves opening and closing. However, the valves of the heart don't finish developing until week 8-9 after fertilization (week 10-11 of pregnancy). That means that in an embryo, we're using the term "heartbeat" in a way that's very different from how we use it in fully developed bodies.

Now, if we revisit the apnea test as an indicator of death, an understanding of this interconnectivity becomes extremely important. Neither the lungs nor the heart function independently. If a person cannot breathe spontaneously, they cannot get oxygen to their blood so even if their heart is still pumping at the time, it's a futile effort. Eventually, as the remaining oxygen is delivered by hemoglobin to the tissue around the body, it will be replaced by carbon dioxide and tissues will start to die from the lack of O_2. At this point, the heart and brain will both stop working if they haven't already.

On the flip side, if a person's heart does not beat, it doesn't matter if they're still breathing because all that oxygen they're taking in doesn't have any way to circulate around the body and the same death will occur.

There are a few ways to combat this. In the case of respiratory failure, we can put someone on a ventilator. In the case of cardiac arrest, we can do chest compressions (artificially pumping the heart by pushing on it) and attempt to get it pumping again with medications and electric shocks. However, the amount of people who survive cardiac arrest to the point they're released from the hospital is currently about 9.3%.[52]

---

[52] American Heart Association. (2023). (rep.). *CARES Annual 2022 Report.* American Heart Association. Retrieved July 6, 2023, from https://mycares.net/sitepages/uploads/2023/2022_flipbook/index.html?page=1.

The chance of someone coming back if their heart stops is, in general, not good.

Why am I describing this? If an embryo has no lungs yet, but does have electrical activity in their heart, they still don't have a functional cardio-respiratory system. Only half of it even exists in any form. According to the definition of death as the lack of a beating heart and spontaneous breathing, we have a non-alive human at this stage.

Also, you'll notice that at the point a heart begins to show electrical pulses, there is no formed brain. Without a brain, we are back to our moral conundrum of life vs. death. If an embryo has electrical impulses from a heart tube, but no brain or lungs, is it alive? It would definitely not pass the apnea test and it would also fail to show having any brain function since it doesn't have a brain at this point.

Everyone has a different answer here, and will continue to make different conclusions throughout this book, but my goal is to make you think about these difficult topics in relation to actual embryonic development. Instead of looking at the whole embryo or fetus at once, think about what's happening in each organ system. There's no single point where we go from "no organ" to "complete organ". Instead, it's a slowly evolving process. Most popular pregnancy sites created for non-medical professionals will note things like "heart starts beating" and "your baby can now move" but those statements can be highly misleading when you look at what's actually happening. The first detectable "heartbeat" comes from pacemaker cells in a tube. Movement is controlled by something only resembling the beginnings of a brain.

Reading a popular website comparing a fetus to the size of a fruit isn't going to cut it if you're trying to argue the nuances of life and embryonic development. However, having a strong understanding of embryology to fall back on will definitely help you in the long run.

Chapter 7

Conception with Help: IVF and Egg Donation

Surprisingly, IVF (the creation of embryos) and abortion (the loss or destruction of them) overlap massively when it comes to the personhood debate. You might have thought we left the topic behind in the pregnancy chapter, but here, again, we have to ask "when does life begin?" Egg retrieval for IVF and egg donation are done with the same medications and procedures, so I'm going to lump them together. What happens after retrieval and how these two processes are regulated introduces both differences and an opportunity for debate.

In terms of egg donation, we see issues popping up regarding the ethics of selling human tissue, custom-made babies and parental rights. For example, when I was in my 20s, I donated eggs in order to pay off some school, medical, and credit card debt. For 17 of my unused eggs, I got a fresh financial start and a family somewhere out there got hand-picked genetic material to make a baby (or babies). The amount of money I made rivaled what I could have brought home working full-time for half a year and it came in a lump sum so I could eliminate interest payments up-front. The United States is unique in this – many countries do not allow eggs to be sold. In America, on the other hand, repeat egg donors can set themselves up for years financially. I once met a woman who paid her full Ivy League PhD tuition with repeat egg donation.

Additionally, donor eggs are often hand-selected based on perceived genetic superiority. The fact that I had multiple relatives who had lived past 90 in my gene pool was a big selling point. Add in an art background, love of writing, and participation in competitive sports, and those eggs were a good fit if someone was hoping for a physically fit, artsy baby. You wouldn't be alone if you thought this type of genetic selection sounds similar to another point in history when the selection of babies for physical and developmental abilities was in vogue.

I'm not saying it's the same, but we can't separate the idea of eugenics entirely from egg selection. After all, buying eggs in the United States is a highly selective practice where intended parents can choose a donor who has the physical traits (perceived beauty, hair color, eye color) they want in their child while eliminating risk factors for genetic disorders, socially undesirable traits (women who are obese, neurodivergent or have a low IQ are typically not accepted as donors.

> ***Paid for eggs?*** Should human eggs and other organs/tissue be treated equally regarding commercial donation?
> In the United States, donating organs for profit is illegal, but getting paid to donate eggs, sperm, and/or plasma is common. American egg donors are usually paid between $5,000 - $10,000. Desirable donors can make over $30,000 per cycle. However, in countries like the UK and France, egg donors do not receive compensation. In Germany, Norway, Switzerland and Turkey, donation is completely banned.
>
> C Calhaz-Jorge and others, Survey on ART and IUI: legislation, regulation, funding and registries in European countries: The European IVF-monitoring Consortium (EIM) for the European Society of Human Reproduction and Embryology (ESHRE), *Human Reproduction Open*, Volume 2020, Issue 1, 2020, hoz044, https://doi.org/10.1093/hropen/hoz044

On the flip side, egg donors give women who don't have viable eggs of their own the ability to have a baby when they otherwise wouldn't be able to.

Problematic genetic selection or miraculous conception – you decide.

The same process egg donors go through is also used to obtain eggs from a person who will then use her own eggs to do in vitro fertilization and transfer embryos back into her own womb.

How does it work?

The goal of egg retrieval for both donation and IVF is to collect multiple mature oocytes from the ovaries. The more oocytes available, the better. While there's no established protocol regarding how many eggs to retrieve, typically 2 is the minimum number a physician wants to remove. The average is somewhere between 8 and 20 with extremes at the higher and lower ends. Considering the massive number of oocytes that die before maturing during monthly cycles, giving up 20+ doesn't make any difference to the health or fertility of most women.

The whole process involves several steps: preparation, stimulation, follicle triggering, and retrieval. While there are multiple medication protocols that can be used, there's a general step-wise approach to getting it done.

Preparation - Birth control may be given a few weeks before menstruation for two reasons. 1. If the eggs will be donated to another person, it allows a physician to sync up donor and recipient cycles. This way, the recipient of the egg will be at the correct point in her ovulatory and menstrual cycles to receive a fertilized embryo for pregnancy. Remember, if we insert an embryo before there's a sufficiently juicy uterine lining, it won't be able to implant. 2. Oral birth control suppresses ovulation and stabilizes the hormones that typically have big swings before, during, and after ovulation. By doing this, fertility specialists are starting with a more controlled environment to alter hormone levels in.

In some cases, a GnRH agonist like leuprolide acetate or Lupron will be given about a week before menstruation. Here's a good example of how pharmacology isn't as simple as one might think. Typically, gonadotropin-releasing hormone (GnRH) comes from the hypothalamus and binds to receptors on the pituitary gland. This binding stimulates the release of LH and FSH which then leads to development of oocytes and, eventually, ovulation with an LH surge.

So, if we want to suppress LH and FSH production and prevent natural ovulation, why would we give a medication that looks like GnRH? Wouldn't that make *more* LH and FSH?

At first, Lupron does cause a spike in FSH and LH levels, but as FSH and LH increase, the body recognizes the artificially inflated levels and goes "woah! We have too much of this!" then reduces production/release of gonadotropins. This results in down-regulation or "pituitary suppression". Basically, by stimulating release of FSH and LH with a GnRH agonist, we cause the levels to spike enough that a long-term *decrease* occurs.

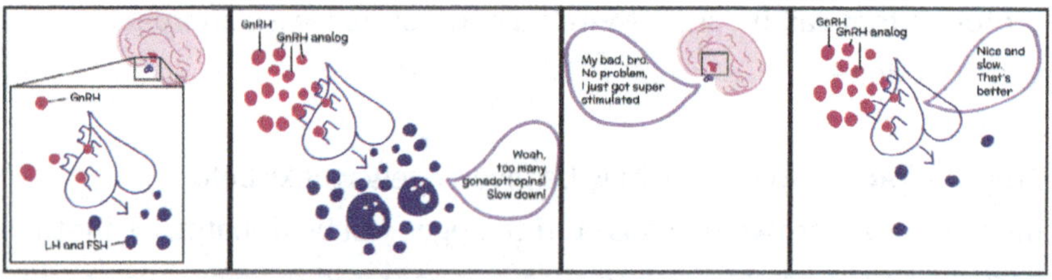

This down regulation continues for the majority of the egg retrieval cycle so that no oocyte matures or pops out on its own. In this process it's not about removing or adding hormones to the cycle, it's about *controlling* the hormones in the cycle. This way, fertility specialists can decide when follicles will mature and release with medication.

Stimulation - Once menstruation occurs (marking day 1 of an egg retrieval/IVF cycle), the focus shifts to stimulating as many follicles as possible to grow simultaneously. To do this, injections of FSH and LH are administered by the patient at home every day.

Despite being totally fine with sticking needles in other people, I personally got hung up on this part of the process when I did it myself. Every night, I'd dance around my bathroom holding a needle, repeatedly attempting to stick myself in the abdomen and then chickening out. A five second task usually took about 20 minutes of my day. But needle sticks are an inevitable part of the egg retrieval process so if someone wants eggs, they're going to need to deal with needles.

If a patient was given a GnRH agonist before starting their cycle, they will continue taking it (remember, control of hormones is the goal; by decreasing the natural production of FSH and LH, a medical professional can control exactly how much is in the system by stimulating or adding those hormones intentionally via injection).

In some women, a GnRh agonist is *not* used pre-menstruation. If that's the case, it's important to make sure LH doesn't surge near the end of the cycle. A natural surge would lead to the loss of all those oocytes that were carefully cultivated. For these patients, a GnRH **ant**agonist is given several days before ovulation/retrieval. The antagonist works opposite to the agonist. When we use antagonists, imagine sticking a bit of bubble gum to the receptor, blocking it from connecting with its matching piece/ligand. In the case of IVF and egg donation, Ganirelix (ganirelix acetate) or Cetrotide (cetrorelix) are typically used for this purpose and block receptors for GnRH so cells are not stimulated to produce an LH surge.

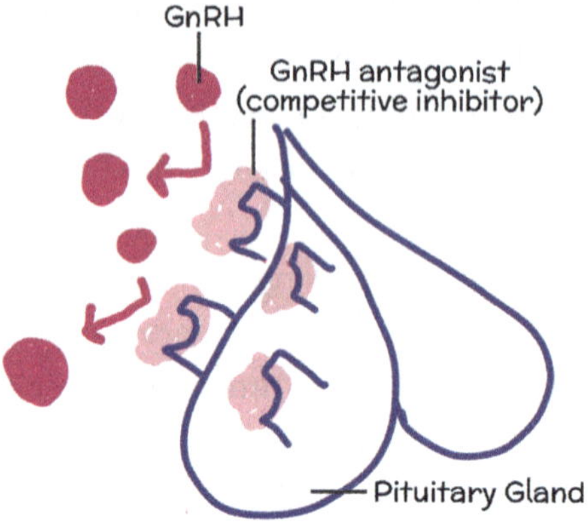

The goal is to get a lot of follicles in both ovaries to about 18 mm. However, it's a very fine line between "enough" and "too much." If the ovaries are overstimulated, follicles may grow too big causing abdominal pain and swelling, as well as dangerous fluid imbalances. Additionally, an ovary that's too full becomes very heavy and can flip itself over causing ovarian torsion. This leads to a lack of blood flow and can cause the death of an ovary. Frequent clinic visits during IVF and egg donation help monitor and prevent these risks.

Trigger - Once ultrasound and hormone levels indicate the follicles are ready for retrieval, an injection of human chorionic growth hormone (hCG) is given. The timing of this is extremely specific. If you've ever donated eggs or done IVF, you'll remember your physician giving you a handout detailing the EXACT TIME to self-administer this medication, possibly with a second reminder from a nurse on your way out, and maybe even a follow-up call that evening. Once hCG is given, it stimulates the final phase of maturation, preparing the oocytes for ovulation. The goal is to collect the eggs right before they are released from the ovaries so they are at their most mature. However, wait too long and they'll be lost to the natural cycle of ovulation and menstruation.

Retrieval - 36 hours after administration of hCG, the oocytes will be retrieved with the help of an internal ultrasound. For anyone who has known a pregnant person (which should be just about every human reading this), an ultrasound is the procedure that spits out those grainy black and white images of babies in utero. An internal version of an ultrasound involves sticking a wand into the vaginal canal to see a similar image of a person's internal structures from another view. The internal ultrasound will guide a large aspiration needle that's passed through the vaginal wall and into the ovaries where fluid containing the oocytes is sucked through the needle, out of the body, and into a collection tube.

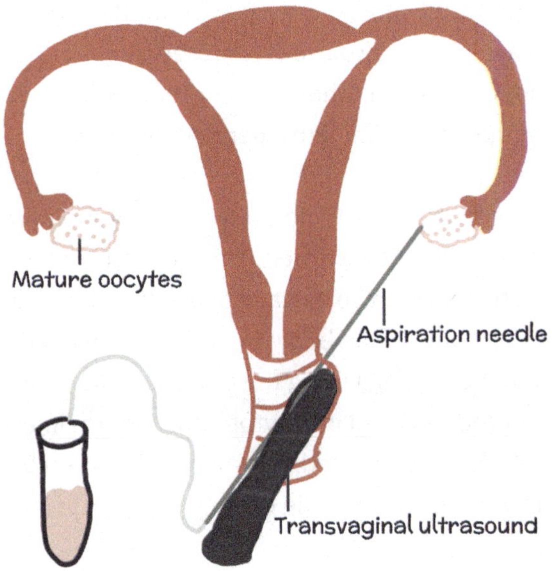

For an egg donor, the job is done. For a person completing an IVF cycle, this is merely the first half of the process. This is where the ethical ambiguity typically begins since now we have eggs outside of the body that may develop into future babies, or may not, depending on what happens next.

Before having them fertilized, retrieved eggs can be frozen for storage in a process called cryopreservation. Because the quality of a person's eggs decreases with age, a person may choose to freeze their eggs while young to reduce any stress related to aging and reproductive health. For example, less than 15% of oocytes in the ovaries of someone in their mid-30s have an incorrect number of chromosomes (referred to as aneuploidy), but that number jumps to over 50% after the age of 40.[53] Eggs with too many, or too few, chromosomes may be completely non-viable, or they may lead to trisomies like Down Syndrome which can come with developmental delays, physical abnormalities including heart defects, low IQ, and a decreased ability to live an independent adult life. If a person chooses to preserve her eggs in her early 20s, she'll be able to use those eggs for IVF at an older age without the stress of oocyte degradation. Many people also use cryopreservation for oocytes retrieved before doing chemotherapy or other medical treatments that may negatively impact or eliminate a person's fertility.

However, if the eggs are going to be used relatively soon for IVF, they are typically fertilized before being frozen. This can happen by squirting sperm onto a petri dish with an egg and allowing fertilization to occur similarly to how it would in the body. Or, if the sperm needs a little help, it can be injected into the egg using the tiniest needle guided by microscope in a process called intracytoplasmic sperm injection (ICSI). Regardless of which option is used, somewhere between 50-70% of eggs will survive fertilization. The rest die off.

Now a person has a bunch of fertilized eggs waiting to be used. What happens next? They can be implanted, frozen, destroyed, tested, donated to research, abandoned, gifted, or fought over.

---

[53] Thomas, C., Cavazza, T., & Schuh, M. (2021). Aneuploidy in human eggs: contributions of the meiotic spindle. *Biochemical Society transactions*, *49*(1), 107–118. https://doi.org/10.1042/BST20200043

Preimplantation Genetic Testing

Before we talk about genetic testing, think about the questions below so you can consider these points while reading ahead.

1. Would you support a family destroying embryos based on sex alone?
2. Should a family be able to select an embryo to be a "Savior Sibling" (the commonly used term for a sibling who has matching tissue and is born to donate bone marrow or blood to a sick older sibling)?
3. If an embryo has genetic markers that may develop into chronic disease, should that embryo be destroyed based solely on those markers?

These aren't just theoretical questions. Preimplantation genetic testing (PGT) allows for all of the above. In a 2020 Assisted Reproductive Technology (ART) report released by the CDC, 16% of families chose to have PGT done before transfer.[54] After an egg is retrieved and fertilized, it develops into a blastocyst around day 5-6. At that point, a few cells are removed from the part of the cell mass that will become the placenta (trophectoderm cells) and are sent for genetic testing. While waiting for results, the embryo will be frozen using cryopreservation for about a week.

Genetic testing results can show the sex of the embryo, if it's a carrier for any single-gene genetic disorders, and/or if it's an HLA (human leukocyte antigen) match for a living relative. Based on the parents' wishes, only embryos with the chosen characteristics will be transferred for implantation.

PGT-M, or preimplantation genetic testing for monogenic disorders, makes a future with children possible for families who have genetic

---

[54] Centers for Disease Control and Prevention. 2020 Assisted Reproductive Technology Fertility Clinic and National Summary Report. US Dept of Health and Human Services; 2022.

disorders in their DNA. For example, cystic fibrosis is an autosomal recessive disease, meaning you need two copies of the affected gene to be symptomatic. People with this disorder typically have lung and GI damage due to mucus buildup and may have a life expectancy nearly 10 years shorter than average.[55] If both parents carry the gene for cystic fibrosis, but are not affected, they may choose to do IVF with PGT-M in order to prevent having an affected child.

While cystic fibrosis requires two copies of the affected gene to be symptomatic, making it an autosomal recessive trait, some diseases are sex-linked. An example of this is hemophilia, a disorder that can cause uncontrolled bleeding. The gene for hemophilia is on the x chromosome, which is the female sex chromosome. Genotypic men have an x chromosome and y chromosome, but females have two x chromosomes. In the case of hemophilia, the affected gene does not produce the proteins needed to properly form blood clots. If a baby boy is born with one y chromosome and an affected x chromosome, he will not make the clotting factors necessary for bleeding management. However, if a baby girl is born with two x chromosomes, and only one is affected, the other chromosome will be enough to tell the body to produce clotting proteins and she will not have the same problems as the affected boy. Because of this, sex selecting embryos that are only female will prevent a couple from having a baby who has hemophilia assuming only the mother carries the altered gene.

---

[55] *Understanding changes in life expectancy*. Cystic Fibrosis Foundation. (n.d.). https://www.cff.org/managing-cf/understanding-changes-life-expectancy

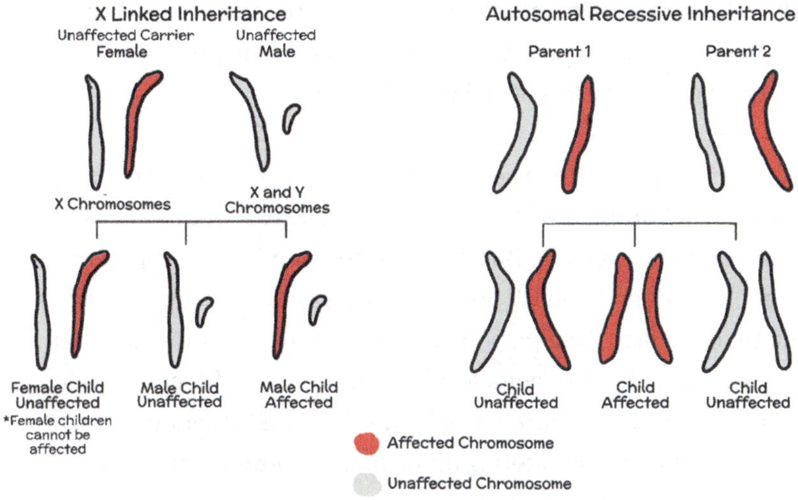

What if a baby already has a blood disorder? In the case of beta thalassemia, there's less hemoglobin in the red blood cells than normal and the blood can't carry enough oxygen and nutrients around the body to keep tissues healthy. In order to keep a person's organs from being damaged by lack of quality blood, these patients may need frequent blood transfusions and/or a bone marrow transplantation. If a family already has a child with severe beta thalassemia, they may want to do two things: 1. Seek PGT-M to ensure a second child does not have the genes for beta thalassemia and 2. Use PTT (preimplantation tissue testing) to have a second child that is a tissue match (HLA match) for the affected child. By having a test for HLA matching done, an embryo can be chosen

> ***Question to Ponder:*** PGT starts a difficult discussion about how the right to life intersects with quality of life. Should embryos be destroyed for disorders that do not limit life expectancy, like deafness? What does that mean for the current and future deaf community if hearing impaired children are never born?
> Should PGT and embryo destruction be subject to the same regulation as genetic testing and pregnancy termination in vivo?

that will be able to donate bone marrow to the first sibling. This is sometimes called a Savior Sibling, and is one of the promoted uses of PGT testing at many fertility clinics.

In the United States, the use of PGT is unrestricted. However, our neighbors in Europe tend to be more cautious with reproductive technology. For example, PGT can only be done for 600 approved genetic disorders in the UK (including the examples of cystic fibrosis and beta thalassemia).[56] If a person has a genetic disorder that's not on the list, they would have to get a fertility clinic to apply for government approval for testing before going forward. This is designed to limit the scope of testing to life-altering monogenic disorders rather than cosmetic or mild abnormalities.

Transfer - Once an egg is fertilized and reaches the blastocyst phase, it's inserted into the uterus via a long plastic tube. Doctors try to time a transfer so it coincides with the period of a female's monthly cycle just after ovulation when the endometrial lining is nice and prime for implantation. From there, we cross our fingers and hope for good outcomes. Out of all transferred embryos, 49.8% will result in a live birth in the United States as of 2020. IVF is not an easy process physically or emotionally. The number of eggs and embryos that fail to become viable pregnancies is significant and the loss at each step can cause a range of emotions from frustration to despair.

Some women try to combat this by requesting the transfer of multiple embryos at once. In fact, for families who attempted IVF years ago, it may have been normal practice for your physician to transfer a whole gaggle of embryos into your uterus at once. According to the CDC, in 2011, only 20.6% of transfers were done as a single embryo transfer as opposed to multiples. In 2020, that percentage rose to 80.4%. Why? The

---

[56] Human Fertilisation and Embryology Authority. (n.d.). *Approved PGT-M and PTT conditions*. HFEA. https://www.hfea.gov.uk/treatments/embryo-testing-and-treatments-for-disease/approved-pgt-m-and-ptt-conditions/

success of IVF transfer has increased, meaning fewer embryos are lost in the transfer process. Additionally, women with multiple embryos transferred were having twins/triplets/etc that they didn't plan for.

If you're as old as I am, you probably remember OctoMom famously having 8 babies after demanding her doctor transfer 12 embryos at once.[57] Not only are 8 babies a lot to care for (I remember when looking for a daycare in NYC, I discovered the legal ratio of adults to babies was 1:4 with no more than 8 infants in a combined group,[58] so having 8 babies for one mom is double the legal ratio), but with every fetus added to a pregnancy, the risks involved in carrying that pregnancy to term rise sharply. Nowadays, the American Society for Reproductive Medicine states that women under 37 should receive a single blastocyst transfer only, and older patients should receive no more than 3 blastocysts at once.[59]

Cryopreservation for later use - If you've ever experienced a Midwestern winter, you know what happens when frozen water expands. Rain falls on a concrete road, small cracks fill up with water. As winter descends upon the land, those small rivers of water freeze and expand, cracking the concrete and causing the potholes that every driver learns to deal with by the time the New Year comes around.

> **Question to Ponder:** When an egg is removed from the ovaries, should it be afforded any more protection than a skin graft or donated cornea?

[57]Popescu, A. (2018, December 15). *The octomom has proved us all wrong*. The New York Times. https://www.nytimes.com/2018/12/15/style/octomom-kids-2018.html

[58] NYC Health. (2019). *What Group Child Care Providers Should Know* . NYC, NY; NYC Health. Retrieved June 23, 2023,.

[59] Practice Committee of the American Society for Reproductive Medicine and the Practice Committee for the Society for Assisted Reproductive Technologies. Electronic address: ASRM@asrm.org (2021). Guidance on the limits to the number of embryos to transfer: a committee opinion. *Fertility and sterility, 116*(3), 651–654. https://doi.org/10.1016/j.fertnstert.2021.06.050

Water in cells acts the same way, if we toss an embryo into freezing temperatures, the crystalized water will expand and burst the cell membrane. Instead, fertilization specialists will use a cryoprotectant to replace the water in the cell.[60] Once this is done, the embryo can be slowly frozen and then stored in tanks of liquid nitrogen at around -321° Fahrenheit (-196.1° Celsius). When the intended parent is ready for transfer, the embryo will be thawed and the cryoprotectants will leave the cell before it's inserted into the uterus.

Disposal - Embryos that are not used can be thawed and then disposed of as medical waste. In one survey of fertility clinics, a group of researchers asked about disposal practices. Out of 703 responses, they found the process varies widely with some practices fulfilling requests for prayer or burial, and others simply disposing of embryos in a trash bin.[61]

In more conservative or religious circles where the practice of destroying embryos is frowned upon, it might be preferable to only create 1-3 embryos in the first place with the intention of using every one. Otherwise, the issue of disposal becomes a problem.

Consider PGT. If a family who is opposed to embryo destruction chooses to undergo IVF and has only 2 embryos created, what happens if one of those embryos ends up having a deadly genetic disorder? It's unlikely

---

[60] Pouria Tirgar, Fatemeh Sarmadi, Mojgan Najafi, Parinaz Kazemi, Sina AzizMohseni, Samaneh Fayazi, Ghazaleh Zandi, Nikta Ziaie, Aida Shoushtari Zadeh Naseri, Allen Ehrlicher, Mojtaba Dashtizad; Toward embryo cryopreservation-on-a-chip: A standalone microfluidic platform for gradual loading of cryoprotectants to minimize cryoinjuries. *Biomicrofluidics* 1 May 2021; 15 (3): 034104. https://doi.org/10.1063/5.0047185

[61]Simopoulou, M., Sfakianoudis, K., Giannelou, P., Rapani, A., Maziotis, E., Tsioulou, P., Grigoriadis, S., Simopoulos, E., Mantas, D., Lambropoulou, M., Koutsilieris, M., Pantos, K., & Harper, J. C. (2019). Discarding IVF embryos: reporting on global practices. *Journal of assisted reproduction and genetics, 36*(12), 2447–2457. https://doi.org/10.1007/s10815-019-01592-w

that anyone will want to accept a donated embryo with a genetic condition. Should the family reconsider its beliefs on embryo destruction? Should they be forced to implant an embryo they know won't survive into adulthood? Or, should PGT be reserved for only those individuals who are willing to destroy and/or donate unwanted embryos to medical research?

Question to ponder: A blastocyst conceived through in vitro fertilization and a blastocyst conceived naturally in the fallopian tube are at the same stage of development. Both were fertilized about 5 days ago, and neither is implanted.
Knowing that, should emergency contraceptive ulipristal acetate (that may [or may not] have post-ovulatory effects) be restricted in states like Louisiana that grant embryos person-hood rights? Should IUDs as emergency contraceptives be allowed?

Most importantly, if these embryos can be disposed of with a good conscience, does that impact one's view on the start or sanctity of life related to abortion? These embryos are at the blastocyst stage of development which occurs during the 2nd week of an in vivo pregnancy (about 6 days after fertilization). As a point of reference, this would be the point that emergency contraceptives like Ulipristal Acetate or an emergency IUD may still be able to prevent implantation of a fertilized egg in the womb.

Again, the moral answers to these questions aren't ones I can answer for you. But the science does tell us what is happening and where in the process an embryo is so we can form more coherent opinions related to when, and when not, embryos should be protected.

Donation - When disposal isn't an option, families can choose to donate embryos to either another family or to medical research. In the United States, it can be tricky to find a donation route for medical research but companies like Reprotech (https://www.reprotech.com/embryo-donation-disposition/) can link the owners of embryos to possible donation sites. Alternatively, a fertility clinic may have research connections they can share with clients on request.

Other organizations help families donate embryos to parents who are also trying to conceive but cannot use their own sperm or eggs for whatever reason. One of the most recognized organizations doing embryo adoption and donation is The National Embryo Donation Center (https://www.embryodonation.org/).

Embryo donation is still relatively uncommon, but it's an option for people with extra embryos who don't mind knowing their genetic offspring is being raised in an unknown family.

Compassionate transfer - For women who feel especially attached to their embryos, the idea of compassionate transfer has been gaining momentum. This involves the same cost and process as a regular blastocyst transfer but instead of transferring the embryo during a fertile period, the transfer is done during a time in the reproductive cycle when it's least likely to implant. Then, the embryo will be flushed out with the rest of her coiled arteries, blood, and tissue, during the woman's monthly period. This can be a good alternative for people who have an emotionally difficult time disposing of embryos, but it comes with a small risk of accidental implantation which could end with an unwanted pregnancy. It also requires both money and time resources (paying for the procedure and having a physician prep and perform the transfer) for an intentionally failed process. Because of that, not every clinic is willing to perform this service.

Abandonment - Surprisingly often, the entire question of disposal goes unanswered since embryos are frequently abandoned by the client. If a facility can no longer contact an individual regarding their embryos or eggs, there's no clear path as to what to do next. One physician, Dr. Craig Sweet, reported to the Associated Press, "About 18 percent, or 300, of his clinic's frozen embryos are abandoned."[62] And that's just a single clinic! There are so many factors that could lead to abandonment: not being able to pay for storage fees, ending a marriage and not assigning responsibility of the embryos in divorce, inability to decide what to do with them, moral upset over destruction, etc. While embryos themselves are tiny, the nitrogen tanks they're stored in are big, and the problem of space is becoming one that fertility clinics need to actively confront.

The In-Between

Imagine undergoing IVF with hopes of starting a family. Shortly after egg retrieval and fertilization, you discover your spouse has been cheating on you despite your being in a monogamous relationship. You cry, scream, grieve; all the feelings that come with betrayal. Then, you move forward with divorce.

As you're splitting up assets, one of you realizes you still have embryos sitting in storage waiting for transfer. You would like to keep them since you still have the same fertility issues that drove you to do IVF in the first place. Your spouse would like them destroyed because they believe having a baby with their genes running around in another family isn't acceptable. Lawyers get involved, custody of the embryos is battled over. Who wins? Who *should* win?

Thankfully, as IVF has become more common, most clinics require an agreement to be signed beforehand stating what will happen in the case of divorce or contested custody. This same agreement likely outlines what will be done with unused embryos regardless of relationship status (do you plan to donate them? Destroy them?).

---

[62] Marchione, M. (2019, January 17). *In limbo: Leftover embryos challenge clinics, couples*. AP NEWS. https://apnews.com/article/health-north-america-us-news-ap-top-news-ca-state-wire-046d6fbc4c564caebac7e560cd87a26a

And this is where the medical procedure of IVF really becomes more of a legal debate. In vitro fertilization itself is usually well understood from a medical perspective by the parents who pursue it, and any arguments to be made usually don't need to be fought "like a doc", but more so "like a lawyer". For example, in the case of unfertilized, frozen eggs, these always remain property of the female who donated them. But what happens with eggs from a separate donor? How about child support? If a divorce occurs and the eggs are used to conceive afterwards, is the genetic father responsible for supporting that child financially?

Outside of legal topics, the issue of embryos and the definition of life remains unchanged. Medically speaking, regardless of its location, an embryo is the same both in vitro and in vivo. Flip-flopping regarding the morality of destroying these embryos based on their location is rarely defensible. If a person believes life starts after fertilization, instead of waiting for a point of viability, that belief should apply to both IVF embryos and in vivo embryos. If a person believes life starts later in fetal development, that definition of non-life should also extend to the fertility lab.

Chapter 8

Abortion: Just the Facts

Recently a tense abortion-centered battle broke out on a popular Facebook group for writers. Someone working on an article asked for sources related to women who have been denied care for ectopic or nonviable pregnancies after the overturn of Roe v. Wade. Another member was quick to point out that treatment for ectopic pregnancies is not, in fact, abortion and is still totally legal. Yet another woman, claimed 'fake news' and within a few minutes, the thread was nearing a hundred comments between essayists, journalists, and freelance writers debating, citing, and cyber-screaming at one another regarding the "truth" surrounding abortion.

These are the people who are writing the stories the rest of us read.

Outside of writing circles, it's the same debate that raged in the comment section of articles about reality star, Jessa Duggar (of *Counting*

On fame, known for her conservative Christian upbringing that very clearly forbids abortion), when she had a D&C after the loss of her baby in utero.[63]

What's so important about a seemingly unimportant Facebook debate or the comment thread surrounding a reality show personality? It shows us that outside of the medical community (and sometimes within it), a huge gap exists in understanding abortion and related procedures. We often fail in even the simplest tasks – agreeing on terminology. Regardless of what side of the argument you fall on, or what part of the discussion you're trying to interpret, abortion is like any other health topic; it's filled with medical-ese and complicated biochemistry that most Americans never came across in school.

Which one of those writers was right and which was wrong? Is treatment for an ectopic pregnancy technically an abortion? Is a nonviable pregnancy that's removed from the womb the same thing as a traditional "abortion"? First, we'll need to cover some basic definitions.

What is an abortion, according to the dictionary?

Abortion, as defined by Merriam-Webster[64] is "the termination of a pregnancy after, accompanied by, resulting in, or closely followed by the death of the embryo or fetus."

Makes sense so far.

Now what about a miscarriage?

If pregnancy naturally fails, the cervix (a small opening at the bottom of the uterus) will open, or dilate, so the contents of the uterus can exit the

---

[63] Etienne, V. (2023, February 27). *Jessa Duggar says she had a D&C, how does that differ from other abortion procedures?*. Peoplemag. https://people.com/health/jessa-duggar-d-and-c-differ-from-other-abortions/

[64] Abortion. 2022. In *Merriam-Webster.com.* Retrieved August 12, 2022, from https://www.merriam-webster.com/dictionary/abortion.

body through the vagina. Most people call this a "miscarriage", but it can also be called a "spontaneous abortion".

An "incomplete miscarriage" is when tissue remains in the uterus even though a miscarriage has begun, and is often referred to as an "incomplete abortion" in medical terms. A "missed miscarriage" or a "missed abortion" is the death of an embryo or fetus in utero *without* the tissue being expelled. In medical terms, miscarriage and abortion are often used interchangeably and with qualifiers.

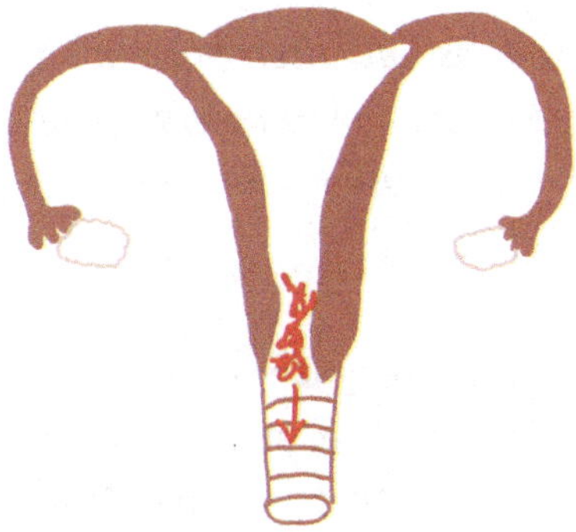

Spontaneous Abortion

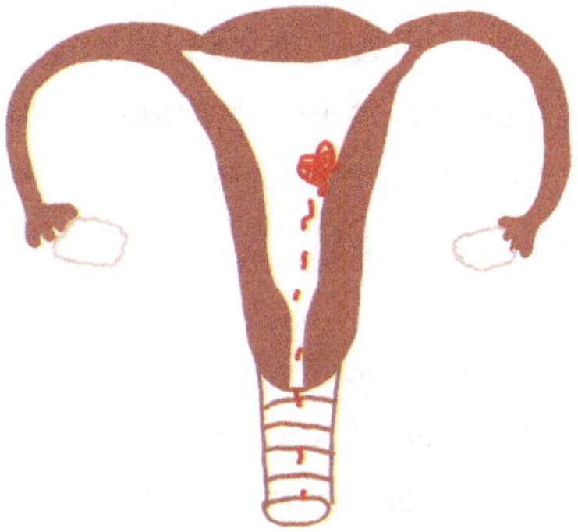

Incomplete Abortion

That's the thing that's tricky about the definition right from the beginning – nowhere in the medical use of the word "abortion" is human intervention specified. A person can have an abortion at a clinic by choice, or can experience a spontaneous abortion at home due to a genetic anomaly.

Already, there are inconsistencies in how the term is used by most people vs. what it actually means.

Abortifacient medications: what are they and how do they work?
What are the procedures used when a medical professional gets involved? First of all, we have abortifacients which are any medications that terminate a pregnancy. To be clear, we're specifically talking about medications that can *cause* an abortion, not the "morning after pill"

which prevents a pregnancy from ever happening in the first place (refer back to chapter 5 if you need a refresher).

Let's start with the abortifacient that started it all: Misoprostol. Misoprostol first entered the scene as a peptic ulcer medication, but it had one extremely unfortunate side effect and that was aborted fetuses. Everyone agreed that we don't want to sacrifice babies in order to heal stomach ulcers, so it's always been restricted for use, or contraindicated if you prefer medical speak, in people who are capable of getting pregnant.

> **Side note: it can still be used as an ulcer prevention medication which brings back the discussion of how/when/if to ban medications that are also used for unrelated conditions.**

How does it work when used to terminate a pregnancy? The same principles we discussed related to birth control are at play here. All of us have little receptors on cells all over our body that pick up different chemicals. When a receptor meets its matching chemical, it triggers some sort of reaction in a cell. Imagine a puzzle piece stuck to the outside of a cell that will only fit with its matching piece. When we make analog medications in a lab, the resulting molecule or compound may not be *exactly* the same as the original, but it's close enough that receptors can't tell the difference. To visualize this, imagine the matching piece might have a little nick in the edge, but it still fits.

Misoprostol looks like prostaglandin E1 (PGE1), a natural chemical in our body, and it's the matching puzzle piece for the PGE1 receptor (no need to remember all these chemical names unless you're taking a biochem exam). When prostaglandins act on your stomach cells, they reduce acid secretions which is why this medication was created as an ulcer treatment. Less acid = less ulcers.

When prostaglandins work on the cells in a person's uterus, something else happens. The cells start contracting until the contents of the uterus are expelled. This is why bodies release a ton of prostaglandins at the end of pregnancy – it causes the uterine muscles to squeeze the baby out of the uterus, into the vaginal canal, and out into the world.

Over time, misoprostol pivoted from an ulcer medication with a bummer of a side effect, to a pill that can be used primarily for abortion. Shortly after, another medication called mifepristone was formulated specifically for blocking or terminating pregnancies and released in the 1980s.[65] Unlike misoprostol, this medication has a totally different mechanism of action, or method, for working.

Instead of acting like a prostaglandin, mifepristone blocks progesterone from working, similarly to how emergency contraceptive pill Ulipristal Acetate acts. Remember, progesterone is released by the corpus luteum and then the placenta to help maintain the pregnancy. When progesterone decreases, the happy environment that's created for baby disintegrates. So mifepristone blocks progesterone, leading to the breakdown of uterine tissue and a host of additional effects like contractions, a softened cervix, and increased sensitivity to prostaglandins (like the ones misoprostol is trying to mimic).

The interesting thing about mifepristone is that it can be used for unrelated diseases and conditions. It happens to block naturally occurring glucocorticosteroids from acting on cells, making it a useful treatment for Cushing's syndrome, a syndrome caused by runaway steroid levels,[66] and can also be used for several types of cancer. Opposite of misoprostol that was designed to treat another condition

---

[65] Institute of Medicine (US) Committee to Study Decision Making; Hanna KE, editor. Biomedical Politics. Washington (DC): National Academies Press (US); 1991. A Political History of RU-486. Available from: https://www.ncbi.nlm.nih.gov/books/NBK234199/

[66] Hopkins, C. (2022, June 25). *The 'abortion pill' may treat a disease affecting many veterans. what happens now?* NBCNews.com. Retrieved August 1, 2022, from https://www.nbcnews.com/health/health-news/abortion-pill-may-treat-dozens-diseases-roe-reversal-might-upend-resea-rcna34812

but is used for abortions, this abortion medication can also be used for other conditions.

Ok, but what does that mean for the patient?
A pregnant person consults a licensed medical professional and is prescribed a dose of misoprostol to take first, then a dose of mifepristone to take within 24-48 hours. Shortly after the second medication, they will experience cramping and bleeding while the contents of the uterus are evacuated. In layman's terms: a person will cramp and bleed until the abortion is complete.

Alternatively, if a patient is experiencing a miscarriage or a miscarriage is imminent, the same medications can help prevent complications and speed up the process. According to ACOG's guide to managing abortion, "within 7 to 10 days, misoprostol showed success rates of 80% to 81% compared with 52% to 85% for expectant management" for early pregnancy loss/miscarriage/spontaneous abortion. The termination of a pregnancy happens *after* the natural death of the fetus. This was the case for our example, Jessa Duggar.

To be clear, a fetus may die or fail to develop due to natural, genetic, or unknown causes *completely unrelated to the parent's health or choices,* and despite that person desperately wanting a baby, the tissue in their uterus will not grow into a living child. A person's body does not always expel the remaining cells and uterine lining on its own, and that's when abortifacient medications are used to clear decaying tissue before it harms the parent.

Merriam Webster would probably classify that as an abortion – would you?

Dilation and curettage
Although the medical procedures above currently account for 54% of

abortions in the United States,[67] most people still think of abortion as an invasive procedure.

The procedure you're probably imagining is one that goes by many names: vacuum aspiration, suction curettage, vacuum D&C. These physical abortions are done with a vacuum which is pretty much what it sounds like – sucking out the contents of the uterus with either a medical style vacuum cleaner or an oversized syringe.

The actual procedure is pretty straightforward. First, a practitioner injects painkilling lidocaine around the cervix (the narrow end of the uterus that opens into the vagina). Then, if the cervix is not dilated enough by use of medication or natural dilation, a dilator is inserted to help. Larger and larger diameter tools are slid into the cervix until it's sufficiently widened. It's kind of like stretching your earlobes if you've ever had piercings.

Once the cervix is wide enough, a cannula is inserted (which is just a fancy word for a tube) and a manual vacuum device is attached to the end of the cannula, leading from the uterus, down the vagina, and outside of the body. In some facilities, an electric vacuum device is preferred. The end result is the same – suction pulls out the contents of the uterus.

In the past, a traditional D&C may have included scraping tissue from the uterus with a sharp tool, but this came with some risk of damage to

---

[67] Jones, R. K., Guttmacher Institute, Nash, E., Cross, L., Philbin, J., & Kirstein, M. (2022, July 14). *Medication abortion now accounts for more than half of all US abortions*. Guttmacher Institute. Retrieved August 1, 2022, from https://www.guttmacher.org/article/2022/02/medication-abortion-now-accounts-more-half-all-us-abortions

the uterine wall.[68] Because of that, many organizations have changed their recommendations to suction procedures only when possible.

What about 2nd and 3rd trimester abortions?

This is where things get more complicated due to regional differences and variations in guidelines. Late-term abortions done over 21 weeks of pregnancy account for less than 1% of abortions in the United States according to the CDC.[69] To phrase that another way, 99% of abortions are "early-term" abortions ("early-term" and "late-term" are not medical terms, but are commonly used in political and public spheres). Even when legal, late-term abortions are not a commonly used procedure.

Of those later-term abortions, 87.0% were performed with surgery or suction and 11.6% were done medically. Medical abortion can still be done using mifepristone and misoprostol with up to 94% efficacy between 12 and 24 weeks of gestation according to a study done in Hawaii,[70] but many practitioners prefer physical procedures after 12-16 weeks, which may help account for the large portion of D&Cs compared to medically managed abortions after the first trimester. If a physical procedure is preferred, it will vary based on the pregnancy, cause of termination, and patient's wishes. One option is that the amniotic fluid can be drained, and the fetus removed using forceps.[71] If a fetus dies in

---

[68] Kakinuma T, Kakinuma K, Sakamoto Y, Kawarai Y, Saito K, Ihara M, Matsuda Y, Sato I, Ohwada M, Yanagida K, Tanaka H. Safety and efficacy of manual vacuum suction compared with conventional dilatation and sharp curettage and electric vacuum aspiration in surgical treatment of miscarriage: a randomized controlled trial. BMC Pregnancy Childbirth. 2020 Nov 16;20(1):695. doi: 10.1186/s12884-020-03362-4. PMID: 33198679; PMCID: PMC7667767.

[69] Kortsmit K, Mandel MG, Reeves JA, et al. Abortion Surveillance — United States, 2019. MMWR Surveill Summ 2021;70(No. SS-9):1–29. DOI: http://dx.doi.org/10.15585/mmwr.ss7009a1

[70] Joensuu-Manninen, H., Kuvaja, P. and Talvensaari-Mattila, A. (2010), Clinical efficacy of mifepristone and misoprostol in second trimester pregnancy termination. Acta Obstetricia et Gynecologica Scandinavica, 89: 1552-1556. https://doi.org/10.3109/00016349.2010.513427

[71] Second-trimester abortion. Practice Bulletin No. 135. American College of Obstetricians and Gynecologists. Obstet Gynecol 2013;121:1394– 1406.

utero, a patient may need to be induced to give birth vaginally which is done with a medication called oxytocin, or a medication we've already talked about: misoprostol.[72]

Because later-term abortions are usually requested due to maternal or fetal complications, the specifics of a case become a lot more important in how these are managed and therefore, are more difficult to discuss as a single entity. To be clear, these are very, very, very rarely (almost never) done by choice due to a baby being unwanted, and in most regions of the world are restricted to medical necessity or genetic abnormality if allowed at all.

In the case of a severe genetic defect, diagnosis might not be confirmed until the second or third trimester which means there's no option for abortion earlier on. In this case, potassium chloride is injected into the fetal heart which causes it to stop beating in under two minutes.[73] Depending on the gestational age of the pregnancy, the fetus may or may not feel pain during this procedure (although it's impossible to know for sure). To minimize potential discomfort, some professionals suggest using fetal analgesia/pain medication.[74]

What is *not* done in the United States are "partial birth" abortions. If you walk past enough anti-abortion protests, you'll eventually see a poster either showing a fetus having its brain removed via suction after the head has been delivered vaginally. Not only was this so rarely performed

---

[72] Kadanali S, Küçüközkan T, Zor N, Kumtepe Y. Comparison of labor induction with misoprostol vs. oxytocin/prostaglandin E2 in term pregnancy. Int J Gynaecol Obstet. 1996 Nov;55(2):99-104. doi: 10.1016/s0020-7292(96)02710-5. PMID: 8960988.
[73] Süzen Çaypınar, S., Oğlak, S.C., Polat, İ. *et al.* A new and more effective feticide technique in late termination of pregnancy: potassium chloride injection into the interventricular septum of the fetal heart. *Arch Gynecol Obstet* 307, 779–787 (2023). https://doi.org/10.1007/s00404-022-06795-8
[74] Senat, M. V., Fischer, C., & Ville, Y. (2002). Funipuncture for fetocide in late termination of pregnancy. *Prenatal diagnosis*, *22*(5), 354–356. https://doi.org/10.1002/pd.290.

that there are no reliable statistics on it, but the act of intentionally causing death to a fetus who has been purposefully delivered was outlawed with the Partial-Birth Abortion Ban Act of 2003.[75]

Fetal reduction with multiples

Strangely, IVF comes under the spotlight again with this one. Especially in the past when multiple embryos were transferred during an IVF cycle, multifetal pregnancy reduction was used as a tool to prevent high risk pregnancies and increase the likelihood of having at least one healthy baby born. The risk of both maternal and fetal complications goes up with the number of fetuses in a pregnancy, so women may choose to remove one or more to protect their own health and/or the health of the remaining baby/babies. While the number of multi-fetus pregnancies has gone up since the use of assisted reproductive technology has become more popular, these same techniques could be used in naturally occurring multiples.

If an embryo or fetus has its own placenta and amniotic sac, potassium chloride (KCl) injection can be used between 11 to 14 weeks of pregnancy just like I mentioned in the previous section.[76] The body will typically absorb the remaining embryonic material so there is no need to remove the fetus.

In the case of monochorionic fetuses, or fetuses sharing a placenta, things get more complicated. Not only are these pregnancies more susceptible to issues like Twin to Twin Transfusion Syndrome because the fetuses are competing for the same source of blood and nutrients, but they're also more difficult to separate since KCl injected into one twin may pass into the other. The most common method for reduction

---

[75] S.3 - 108th Congress (2003-2004): Partial-Birth Abortion Ban Act of 2003. (2003, November 5).
https://www.congress.gov/bill/108th-congress/senate-bill/3

[76] Beriwal, S, Impey, L, Ioannou, C. Multifetal pregnancy reduction and selective termination. *The Obstetrician & Gynaecologist* 2020; 22: 284– 292.
https://doi.org/10.1111/tog.12690

in these cases involves interrupting the blood supply of the umbilical cord for the fetus who will be reduced. This can be done with radiofrequency ablation (using radiofrequency to heat up a tip of a needle that is applied to the umbilical cord), laser ablation, or cautery of the umbilical cord.

And lastly, the ectopic pregnancy.
Ectopic pregnancies are not viable. However, these are also *not* treated in the same way that a typical abortion during an average pregnancy is.

If an embryo starts growing in a fallopian tube and we give a patient abortifacient medications, the uterus will contract (unrelated, you'll produce less stomach acid), and progesterone won't be able to maintain the uterine conditions for pregnancy.

However, the embryo is not in the uterus in an ectopic pregnancy, so none of those solutions will help.

In fact, misoprostol and mifepristone are contraindicated in ectopic pregnancies.[77] Instead, providers use methotrexate, a cancer and arthritis medication. This medication can prevent cells, like those in an embryo – or those in cancer – from replicating correctly. This causes the embryo to stop growing. Surgery can then be used to remove the embryo from wherever it has implanted.

To summarize, in an ectopic pregnancy, the methods are different but the result is still "the termination of a pregnancy after, accompanied by, resulting in, or closely followed by the death of the embryo or fetus."

---

[77]Debnath J, Gulati SK, Mathur A, Gupta R, Kumar N, Arora S, Krishna RB. Ectopic pregnancy in the era of medical abortion: are we ready for it? Spectrum of sonographic findings and our experience in a tertiary care service hospital of India. J Obstet Gynaecol India. 2013 Dec;63(6):388-93. doi: 10.1007/s13224-013-0459-2. Epub 2013 Aug 14. PMID: 24431685; PMCID: PMC3889275.

What does this all mean?

Before declaring verbal war on your friends and family when abortion rights come up, I suggest we all take a moment to think about our own positions without the pressure of an argument.

The common use of the word "abortion" is unspecified and loaded with moral judgment. In the writers' group I'm in, it was one person's opinion that an abortion was specifically the act of a doctor ending a pregnancy with medication, surgery, or a vacuum procedure. A medical professional and health writer pointed out that miscarriages are, medically speaking, "abortions". A parenting writer pointed out that medications used for a missed miscarriage, a.k.a. a "missed abortion", are the same as those used for an elective abortion.

At the end of the debate, everyone is right. It *is* all abortion.

Which is why it's so important to become more nuanced. Let's all take a moment to do better in our discussions, to form more considered opinions. Do you support the use of abortifacient medications? What if used for unrelated ailments like ulcers and cancer? Do we allow vacuum aspirations? How about in the case of a fetus who has already died?

These are the real discussions that need to be had. Not just another argument regarding the legality of a word that's often defined incorrectly anyways.

Chapter 9

The Complications that Complicate Discussion of Pregnancy

For families who have experienced pregnancy complications and/or loss, this chapter may be difficult to read. I'll present the information as medically as possible, but the mention of pregnancy or post-birth loss is unavoidable. While there are some comparisons I'll use to help clarify what's happening at a micro level, I'd like to be clear that despite any silliness, the real world impact of these complications is heartbreaking and life-altering. There is no way a person who has not experienced pregnancy loss can ever understand the soul shattering experience of having to decide between a mother and baby's life, or the deep sadness that sits with a person for the remainder of their years when they've lost a baby.

> If not pregnant, it may be easy to brush off a non-viable pregnancy as a non-event. However, the act of carrying any type of pregnancy, building one's hopes upon the idea of family, and then losing the possibility of that future is a loss that can be felt on a primal, emotional, level that may never go away.
> To all of you who have suffered this devastating travesty, my heart goes out to you. To those of you who haven't, I ask you to discuss these topics delicately in public as you never know who has dealt with them.

To clarify a term commonly used when discussing pregnancy and abortion, a "viable" fetus is one that is capable of living outside of the uterus. A "viable pregnancy" allows a fetus to develop to a point of "fetal viability" (survivability outside the womb). While "viable" will often come with a qualifier like "most likely not–" or "possibly viable with intervention," the opposite word "non-viable" is usually used in absolutes. An ectopic pregnancy is non-viable. A completely molar pregnancy is non-viable. There is no chance of these developing into a baby that can survive.

More than anything, this chapter is really meant to help determine where there is a gray area for ethical and moral debate, and where there is none. I'll cover the most common pregnancy complications, placental issues, and genetic disorders that are brought up in both genetic testing debates (i.e. during IVF or healthy pregnancies) and abortion (when should an exception be made to terminate a pregnancy). But there are thousands of examples, if not tens of thousands, that I will not cover here for lack of space and time.

Chemical pregnancy

This type of pregnancy is really only discussed if a person suspects she lost a pregnancy in the first few weeks. It doesn't cause further complications nor does it require intervention. In fact, up until home pregnancy tests were advertised in 1978, women often didn't know they were pregnant until they were well past the date of their expected period or visibly started to show.[78] Pregnancy loss in the first few weeks almost always went unnoticed and unconfirmed since it's nothing more than a later-than-usual period. In the 1990s, home pregnancy tests became more accurate, and now ClearBlue's Early Pregnancy Detection Test claims to show positive results 6 days before a person's first missed period,[79] which is about 8 days after ovulation. If someone took one of these tests, they'd know they were pregnant well before historical averages. If a person then lost that pregnancy shortly after implantation, they would be aware of it in a way they weren't in previous times.

Unless someone is monitoring her monthly cycles very closely, as is the case in fertility treatments, a chemical pregnancy is still uncommon to catch. Assisted Reproductive Technology (ART) is the main reason we have *any* data on these pregnancies since fertilized eggs are closely tracked during the IVF process. One study found that nearly 25% of all pregnancies fail before being noticed.[80] This could be due to chromosomal abnormalities, low hormone levels, or a million other factors. Again, it's important to remember that events in vitro (out of body) and in vivo (in body) are not always the same. While we can assume there are similar rates of failure in vivo, that may or may not be true.

Blighted ovum or anembryonic pregnancy

The term "blighted ovum" has fallen out of fashion but some women may recognize it over the more recent "anembryonic" or "empty gestational sac" pregnancies. Anembryonic is the most accurate since

---

[78] U.S. Department of Health and Human Services. (n.d.). *Pregnancy test - a thin blue line the history of the pregnancy test - office of NIH history and Stetten Museum*. National Institutes of Health. https://history.nih.gov/display/history/Pregnancy+Test+-+A+Thin+Blue+Line+The+History+of+the+Pregnancy+Test

[79] Clearblue. (2023, May 2). *When can I take a pregnancy test?*. Clearblue. https://www.clearblue.com/pregnancy-tests/early-pregnancy-testing

[80] Annan, J. J., Gudi, A., Bhide, P., Shah, A., & Homburg, R. (2013). Biochemical pregnancy during assisted conception: a little bit pregnant. *Journal of clinical medicine research*, *5*(4), 269–274. https://doi.org/10.4021/jocmr1008w

this is a pregnancy without ("an-") an embryo. An egg will still implant in the uterus but it doesn't develop correctly. This is *not* a future baby.

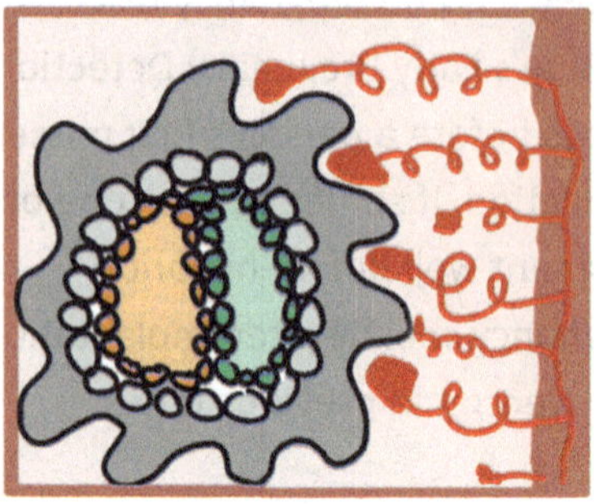
Typical pregnancy during implantation

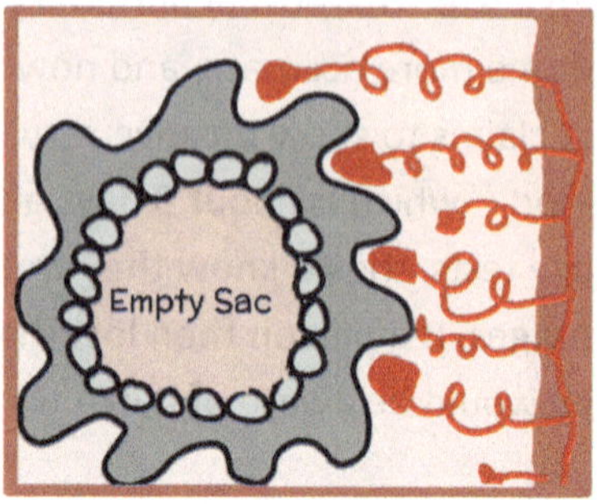

Blighted Ovum or Anembryonic pregnancy

If you refer back to our drawing of a blastocyst, you'll see an inner cell mass/embryoblast and an outer cell mass/ trophoblast. In an anembryonic pregnancy, the trophoblast exists, but the inner cell mass never develops. Because there is still a trophoblast, a syncytiotrophoblast still develops from that layer as implantation occurs and hCG is produced, leading to positive pregnancy tests. During the first ultrasound, instead of a visible embryo there will only be an empty sac.

This will never turn into a fetus and will usually spontaneously abort if left alone. Once discovered, parents may choose to engage in "watchful waiting" which allows the sac to abort naturally, or use misoprostol to cause the uterine contents to evacuate sooner.[81] For patients who are experiencing complications, a D&C is preferred to immediately remove the tissue.

Molar pregnancy (gestational trophoblastic disease)
NPR recently shared a story about a woman in Oklahoma who was

[81] Chaudhry K, Tafti D, Siccardi MA. Anembryonic Pregnancy. [Updated 2023 May 22]. In: StatPearls [Internet]. Treasure Island (FL): StatPearls Publishing; 2023 Jan-. Available from: https://www.ncbi.nlm.nih.gov/books/NBK499938/

denied treatment for a molar pregnancy that had become cancerous.[82] Under abortion law in 2023, it was unclear if the tissue could be removed unless the woman's life was actively threatened (i.e. her vital signs were unstable, she was experiencing shock or blood loss, she was unconscious, etc.). But what is a molar pregnancy? When does a pregnancy become cancerous? Is there any hope of a baby resulting?

Gestational trophoblastic disease (GTD) is typically referred to as molar pregnancy with two types: complete and partial hydatidiform moles. Outside of medical texts, these are mostly just referred to as molar pregnancies with partial and complete moles. A pregnancy becoming cancerous is a later stage progression of GTD.

Complete mole - This mole is **complete**ly molar (or at least that's how I remembered it for exams). Completely molar, meaning no fetus. One of the ways for this to happen is when two sperm fertilize an egg that has no DNA. This leads to two sets of DNA, but they're both coming from the father. Alternatively, one sperm might enter an egg with no DNA and then divide, resulting in the same duplicate set of sperm DNA.

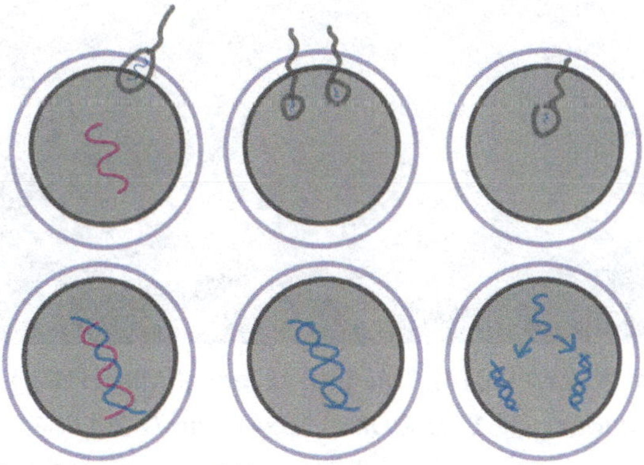

Typical egg + sperm = 1 set of maternal chromosomes and 1 paternal | Empty egg + two sperm = 2 sets of paternal chromosome | Empty egg + one sperm that divides = 2 sets of paternal chromosomes

[82] Simmons-Duffin, S. (2023, April 25). *In Oklahoma, a woman was told to wait until she's "crashing" for abortion care*. NPR. https://www.npr.org/sections/health-shots/2023/04/25/1171851775/oklahoma-woman-abortion-ban-study-shows-confusion-at-hospitals

We still have 46 chromosomes in the resulting cell (2 sets of 23, just like the rest of the cells in our bodies) but this double set of paternal chromosomes causes the syncytiotrophoblast layer to start growing uncontrolled and an embryo never develops. All the chorionic villi that normally grow into the uterus and form the placenta instead fill with fluid and start pumping up like the Hulk in a fit of rage. Those puffed-up villi look similar to a bunch of grapes since their thin membranes resemble grapeskin, and if you were to view one of these pregnancies on ultrasound, you'd see a bunch of fuzz – we call this a "snowstorm appearance".

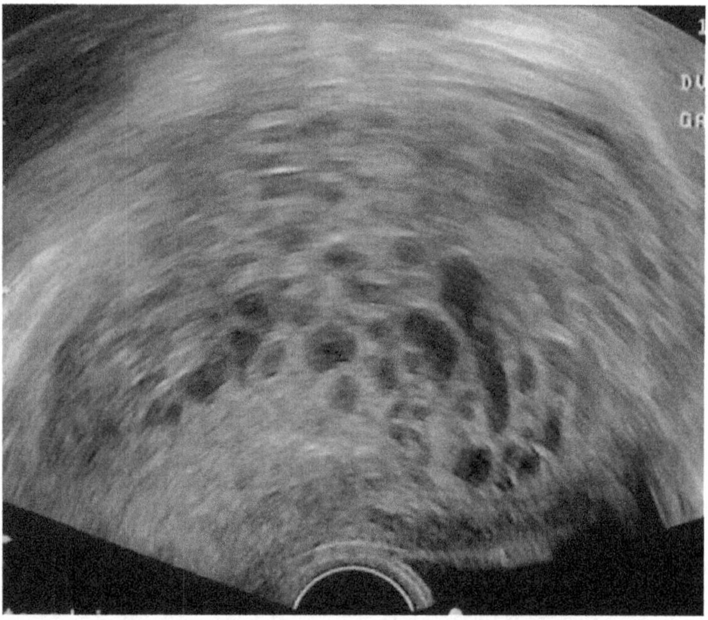

Häggström, Mikael (2014). "Medical gallery of Mikael Häggström 2014". *WikiJournal of Medicine* **1** (2). DOI:10.15347/wjm/2014.008. ISSN 2002-4436. Public Domain

Because this process is driven by syncytiotrophoblast cells, a *ton* of hCG is produced. If you remember from the conception and pregnancy section, normal morning sickness happens when hCG is released after implantation. When an excessive amount of hCG is rapidly produced in a complete mole, women may experience hyperemesis gravidarum which is morning sickness x10,000 and it can cause a person to vomit so much they end up in the hospital for severe dehydration. Additionally, the increase in hormones can stimulate cells outside of the reproductive tract leading to hyperthyroidism, and inside the reproductive system causing more oocytes in the ovaries to mature.

If someone is found to have a complete molar pregnancy, physicians will do a D&C and then prescribe a reliable contraception like oral birth control pills. The second step is imperative because these moles have the highest risk for gestational trophoblastic neoplasm (neoplasm = cancer) with around 15%-20% becoming malignant. To monitor for cancerous growth in the future, a person will have their hCG levels taken every month for six months after the molar pregnancy is resolved. Another spike in hCG means neoplasm. If another pregnancy occurs, hCG levels will also rise, making it impossible to monitor accurately for cancer, which is why it's important to prevent pregnancy during this time.

Since there's a slightly increased risk for repeat molar pregnancies, older women may be offered a hysterectomy as part of treatment. No uterus, means no chance for neoplasm or additional molar pregnancies.

Partial mole - This one is only partial, meaning it may have parts of an embryo or fetus. This typically happens when two sperm enter a normal oocyte. Instead of the desired 2 sets of chromosomes (46 chromosomes in total), we end up with three (69 in total). This type of fertilization will not result in a viable pregnancy or a full-term baby, and if not diagnosed, it will usually spontaneously abort by the second trimester. Despite not being viable, a pregnancy loss later in pregnancy can be deeply traumatic to the family.

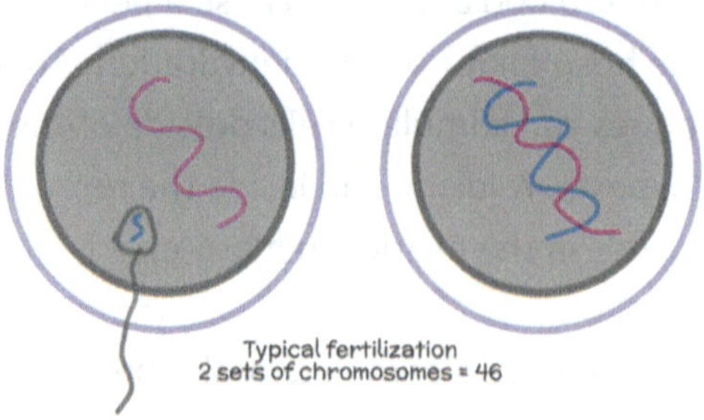

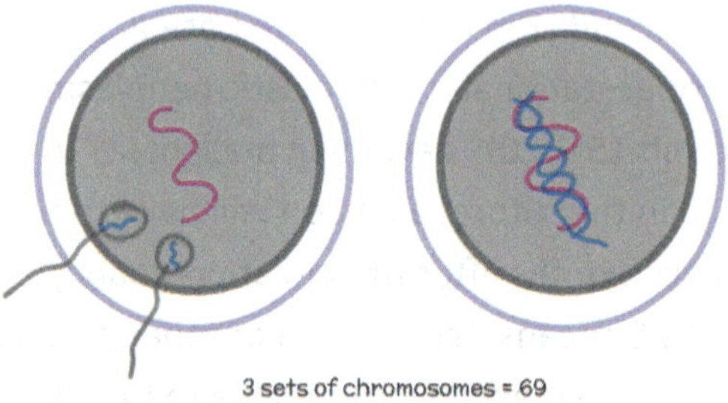

These moles are made up of hydropic villi (overfilled villi), but they have some regular villi mixed in (because these pregnancies are only *partially* molar). In this situation, the overgrowth happens from the cytotrophoblast cells which do not produce hCG, and will grow much slower. These pregnancies may feel normal at first, and in some cases, there will even be electrical flutters detected in the fetal mass resembling a heartbeat. However, as time goes on, an ultrasound will show the same snowstorm image as described above and it will become clear that this is a non-viable pregnancy. Like a complete mole, a D&C will be suggested with oral contraceptives given afterwards to monitor for neoplasms.

Gestational Trophoblastic Neoplasm (cancer)
After a molar pregnancy is removed, hCG levels will drop. If these levels start to increase again in subsequent lab work, we have a problem. This is indicative of gestational trophoblastic neoplasm (GTN) and can happen after any molar pregnancy with the highest risk found in complete molar pregnancies. GTN can also happen after spontaneous abortions, elective abortions, or the live birth of a healthy baby.

Basically, anytime implantation has occurred, it's possible for a person to end up with GTN. But it's rare, so if you happen to be the owner of a fertile uterus, this is *not* one of the many things you should worry about.

GTN shows up in two ways: invasive moles which only grow locally, or choriocarcinoma which can grow quickly and spread to other organs.

Invasive moles - These are very similar to complete and partial moles, but grow into the myometrium (the muscular layer in the uterus, below the stratum basalis) and may metastasize to the lungs[83] or other organs. Treatment is usually methotrexate which inhibits DNA synthesis, preventing cell replication, and has a 100% cure rate in less severe cases. That's a proper cure rate, not just remission.

Choriocarcinoma - This can happen after gestational trophoblastic disease but 25% of all choriocarcinomas come after live births. These cell masses are fast-growing with syncytiotrophoblasts and cytotrophoblasts. A low-risk choriocarcinoma is one that only spreads in the uterus and genital tract. It can be cured with methotrexate 95%+ of the time. A high-risk choriocarcinoma is one that spreads to other body parts, often the lungs, which can result in a patient coughing up blood or having difficulty breathing (needless to say, if you are ever coughing up blood, the first thing you should do is visit an emergency room regardless of if you have a uterus or not). High-risk findings will need to be treated with a range of chemotherapeutic drugs but can still be fully cured 50-75% of the time.

The woman with the cancerous pregnancy

A D&C and/or medical abortion with methotrexate (to stop growth of the tissue) and misoprostol (to help expel it) is the standard treatment for the removal of any pregnancy that is either non-viable or harmful to the mother. In the case of the woman from Oklahoma, assuming she

---

[83] Aminimoghaddam, S., & Maghsoudnia, A. (2017). Unusual Presentation of Invasive Mole: A Case Report. *Journal of reproduction & infertility, 18*(1), 205–209.

had a molar pregnancy, a mass of tissue was growing into something that would never become a baby, possibly invading her uterine tissue. Regulation of elective abortions prevented medical staff from treating her because it may have put them on the wrong side of the law. Instead of getting the medical procedure she needed for a diagnosable condition, she was encouraged to wait until complications arose. Like so many topics in this book, I cannot stress enough how regulations made by people without a deep understanding of disease pathology and related conditions will always have collateral damage. The only thing we can do to help safeguard against that is to make sure the people passing laws understand the wider implications of those laws, not just related to the immediate debate. Almost no medical procedure or medication is used for a single purpose alone and by regulating it for one purpose, all the unrelated patients in need may find themselves without access.

Ectopic pregnancy

In a 2019 version of Ohio bill, HB413, introduced by representatives Candice Keller and Ron Hood, it was written that physicians had to "...[attempt to] reimplant an ectopic pregnancy into the women's uterus". At the time, this was a medically impossible feat.

As of writing this book, this remains a medically impossible feat.

Instead, physicians want to treat these as quickly and definitively as possible, not sit around twiddling their thumbs and considering future innovation. Ectopic pregnancies kill mothers. Plain and simple. One researcher did a review of past medical literature and found that in 1880, 72–90% of ectopic pregnancies resulted in maternal death.[84] That number dropped to 0.14% in 1990 (notice the period BEFORE the number 1, that's just over a tenth of 1 percent!). Modern medicine turned a death sentence into a relatively routine procedure. To put that

---

[84] Lurie S. (1992). The history of the diagnosis and treatment of ectopic pregnancy: a medical adventure. *European journal of obstetrics, gynecology, and reproductive biology*, *43*(1), 1–7. https://doi.org/10.1016/0028-2243(92)90235-q

into perspective, pancreatic cancer is said to have a mortality rate above 90%. Imagine if we suddenly invented a way to drop that to well under 1%. The Nobel Prizes would be lined up, the medical community would be in a state of celebration. Yet we've done that for ectopic pregnancies, and instead of awe and amazement, the debate about how doctors treat these continues to pop up in public spheres on a regular basis.

> ***Prevention:*** Women with a history of untreated STIs have a higher risk for ectopic pregnancies, preterm labor, and infertility. Their babies may have low birth weight, long term developmental delays, blindness, and more.
>
> According to the CDC "congenital syphilis cases have more than tripled in recent years, with more than 2,000 cases reported in 2021 alone." Pregnant women are now passing syphilis to their children at rates much higher than we've seen since 1994.
>
> Think access to sexual health clinics like Planned Parenthood doesn't matter? One solution to decrease pregnancy complications and abortions is to increase access and remove costs associated with preventative care, STI testing/treatment, birth control, and sex education.
>
> Centers for Disease Control and Prevention. (2023, April 11). *STD facts - congenital syphilis*. Centers for Disease Control and Prevention. https://www.cdc.gov/std/syphilis/stdfact-congenital-syphilis.htm#:~:text=What%20is%20congenital%20syphilis%20(CS,Learn%20more%20about%20syphilis.

Let's delve into the anatomy here so there's no confusion. An ectopic pregnancy is a fertilized egg that implants somewhere it doesn't belong. The majority of these pregnancies will end up in the fallopian tubes, implanting before the embryo makes its way to the uterus. For the sake of covering my bases, these *can* implant elsewhere. I found one article that compiled different case reports of unusual implantation sites including the cervical canal, the colon, and an ovary.[85] If you're curious about the many ways fertilized eggs can get lost in the system, then I

---

[85]Badr, Sanaa & Ghareep, Abdel-Naser & Abdulla, Lamya & Hassanein, Rabei. (2013). Ectopic pregnancy in uncommon implantation sites. The Egyptian Journal of Radiology and Nuclear Medicine. 44. 121–130. 10.1016/j.ejrnm.2012.10.006.

suggest reading the original; it's not too heavy on medical terminology and will give you a peek into the world of medical case reports.

To summarize, here are some places doctors have found ectopic pregnancies:

- Ovary - While extremely rare, occasionally an egg will become fertilized in the ovary. One group of researchers were able to show sperm that had ascended the uterus, swum through the fallopian tubes, and entered the ovaries to fertilize an oocyte before it was released.[86] The typical process involves fertilization in the fallopian tubes since sperm cannot normally enter the ovaries (otherwise we'd have thousands of these), but some fluke in the system might explain the rare ovarian pregnancy. I'm going to say this one more time so you don't look silly in a discussion: in a typical female, sperm does **not** enter the ovaries.
  Knowing that, other physicians have suggested that even in rare cases, fertilization in the ovary is impossible. Instead, the fertilized egg travels backwards from the fallopian tube into the ovary (reflux of the egg into the ovary) on a rare occasion. If a fertilized embryo develops in the ovary, it will eventually burst the entire thing, destroying the ovary in the process and causing potentially fatal hemorrhage. These pregnancies are in no way viable. Treatment usually involves surgery, with conservative methods like ovarian wedge resection (where a wedge of the ovary is removed) or complete removal of the ovary.[87] With minimal removal of the ovarian tissue in a wedge resection, women will experience little, if any, loss of fertility.

---

[86] Nada, Z. M., Assaf, N. F., Dubey, S. K., & JMC Board (2005). Human sperm can fertilize ova inside the Graafian follicles before ovulation. *Fertility and sterility, 83*(2), 457–461. https://doi.org/10.1016/j.fertnstert.2004.09.013

[87] Scutiero, G., Di Gioia, P., Spada, A., & Greco, P. (2012). Primary ovarian pregnancy and its management. *JSLS : Journal of the Society of Laparoendoscopic Surgeons, 16*(3), 492–494. https://doi.org/10.4293/108680812X13462882736385

- Abdominal - This one kind of throws the whole anatomy chapter into disarray. How does a fertilized egg find itself outside of the reproductive system?! And if that can happen, can sperm from anal sex fertilize an egg in the fallopian tubes? Can girls pee out of their vaginas?!
  ... no.
  The anatomy still works out. The reproductive system is a generally closed system. Primarily, abdominal pregnancies happen secondary to other pregnancies going wrong. For example, an ectopic pregnancy in an ovary or fallopian tube may rupture allowing the fertilized egg to implant within the abdominal cavity. Similarly, a uterine scar may present a weak spot in a typical uterine pregnancy and allow the fertilized egg to burrow into the abdomen. In terms of preventative medicine, in regions where STIs go untreated there may be women who have enough damage to the fallopian tubes that eggs can escape.[88] (Side note - this is another reason to promote STI education and easy access to reproductive healthcare. Neurosyphilis – or psychiatric illness caused by syphilis – isn't the only thing that can go wrong with untreated disease. There's also an increased risk of Pelvic Inflammatory Disease, pregnancy complications, and infertility). Treatment of abdominal pregnancies is surgery, but there's no single procedure since these pregnancies are a bit of a wild card. You never know what you're going to get so you need a good surgeon to help formulate a personalized plan.
- Cervix - True cervical pregnancies, not just low-lying uterine implantations, are rare. When they happen, it's treated with methotrexate to prevent growth and then removal of the embryonic tissue if needed. If cervical pregnancies are not found early, they carry a huge risk of massive hemorrhage and

[88] Hajji, A., Toumi, D., Laakom, O., Cherif, O., & Faleh, R. (2020). Early primary abdominal pregnancy: Diagnosis and management. A case report. *International journal of surgery case reports*, *73*, 303–306. https://doi.org/10.1016/j.ijscr.2020.07.048

may need to be treated with a complete hysterectomy (removing the uterus). By arguing about the delay of treatment or withholding medications that are primarily used for abortion in this case, a person would not be protecting the rights of the baby inside the cervix (this embryo will never become a viable fetus since it will burst through the cervix first), and instead would be arguing for the loss of all future babies that woman may carry if/when her cervix rips apart and needs to be removed.

The key to preventing future fertility loss in ectopic pregnancies is early detection. By having a skilled sonographer recognize exactly where an embryo is (which can be surprisingly tricky), we can save the lives of countless women.

Hypertension, pre-eclampsia and eclampsia

What does high blood pressure have to do with pregnancy? Besides being one of the most common pregnancy complications, it can threaten the life of both baby and mom. If high blood pressure is diagnosed before 20 weeks of pregnancy, we call it chronic hypertension, meaning it was probably a problem before pregnancy, will continue to be afterwards, and can be managed with hypertensive medications approved for use in pregnancy including hydralazine, labetalol, and nifedipine. If a person is diagnosed with hypertension after 20 weeks, it's usually the result of gestational (pregnancy-related) causes.

On the surface, this doesn't seem like such a big deal. Around half of Americans (47% according to the CDC[89]) are living with hypertension. Who cares?

---

[89] Centers for Disease Control and Prevention. (2023, May 15). *Facts about hypertension*. Centers for Disease Control and Prevention. https://www.cdc.gov/bloodpressure/facts.htm#:~:text=Nearly%20half%20of%20adults%20in,are%20taking%20medication%20for%20hypertension.

To understand when this run-of-the-mill medical problem becomes something more serious, it's important to understand the stages of gestational hypertension. If a pregnant person's systolic blood pressure (top number) is over 140 or the diastolic blood pressure (bottom number) is over 90, it's **high blood pressure/hypertension**. When those numbers go over 160 systolic or 110 diastolic, a pregnant person may experience organ damage, which can lead to proteinuria (peeing out proteins) if it happens to the kidneys. This is when hypertension becomes **"pre-eclampsia"** in the pregnant patient.

Eventually, extremely high blood pressure can lead to maternal blood vessels leaking and causing edema (fluid build-up in the tissues). Imagine if you poked a bunch of holes in the side of a hose – it would still work but it'd leak water in the dirt nearby and everything would get a bit soggy. That's just like our bodies, when the vessels become leaky, fluid squishes into the tissues nearby. This fluid can build up in the lungs (pulmonary edema) or the brain (cerebral edema). There's not much extra space in our skulls, so when our brains get soggy and swell up, things go wrong quickly. Seizures can eventually lead to a coma or death.

In this case, "seizure" is the key word since a patient who has pre-eclampsia, graduates to **"eclampsia"** with the occurrence of a seizure.

Eclampsia is a medical emergency.

Why does it happen? While medicine hasn't definitively explained the cause of gestational hypertension in all cases, we know it's more likely to happen in a first pregnancy and in people 35 years of age or older. Possibly, arteries in the placenta are fibrotic, or more rigid than usual, which causes narrowing of the blood vessels going into and out of the placenta. Because the tubes delivering blood are smaller than usual, pressure builds up behind them, causing an increase in pressure throughout the maternal vascular system. It can also lead to a decrease of nutrient-rich blood reaching the fetus since there's a backup on the maternal side. In more severe cases, the placenta might tear apart from the uterus (placental abruption), which we'll talk about in the next section.

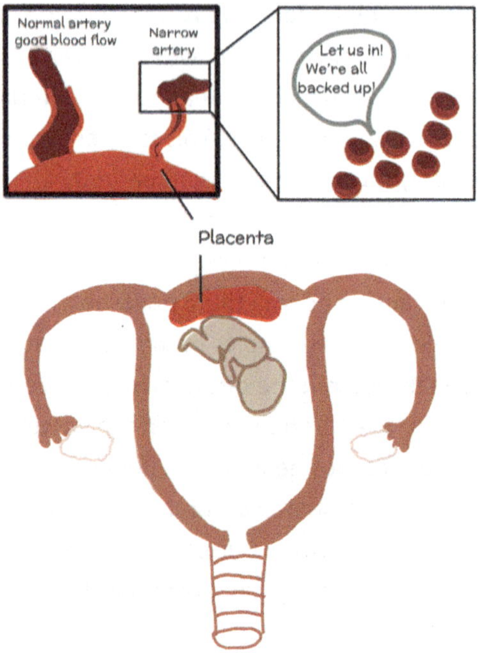

Now, tiny injuries along the maternal blood vessels due to the increase in pressure may start to appear. When blood vessels are injured, one of the first things that happens is pieces of cells called platelets come and stick to the injury, launching a very complicated, infinitely long cascade of events that eventually causes coagulation and building a clot at the site of injury to prevent blood from spilling out. This cascade of events is powered along by little proteins called clotting factors, and if you ever want to feel the pain of a first- or second-year medical student, go and memorize each individual step, enzyme, protein and reaction in this cascade. It's the academic version of bamboo shards under the fingernails.

These tiny little clots along the vessel walls are also known as "thrombi." Think of the thrombi as little dollops of glue inside a hose covering a bunch of itty-bitty leaks. When red blood cells come charging down that same blood vessel, they run into the clots and burst apart. Welcome to "hemolysis" (lysis means "rupture", and hemo refers to the blood).

Imagine this: the narrow blood vessels reduce the amount of blood going to the liver, causing liver damage, platelets are all busy stuffing up tiny endothelial injuries in the blood vessels, and hemolysis is happening. This constellation of events is called HELLP, which stands for "hemolysis," "elevated liver enzymes" (from liver damage) and "low platelets."

Second trimester abortion exception?

Pre-eclampsia is determined by high blood pressure and proteinuria. It's most often diagnosed in the third trimester and can be treated effectively with medication in most cases. However, if it's found early in the second trimester, the likelihood of life-threatening complications is much higher. If eclampsia (high blood pressure, protein in the urine, and the addition of seizures) appears before the end of the second trimester, abortion may become the only realistic option as the fetus is not yet viable and eclampsia can only be cured with delivery.

Would you support an abortion in the second trimester for cases of eclampsia? What medical facts from this section support your belief?

Even worse than HELLP is disseminated intravascular coagulation (DIC, pronounced as the letters, not a single word, even though it's more fun to read it all together). DIC is not something you want to have happen to you. 47%-57% of people who are diagnosed with DIC will die.[90] Because all the clotting factors are off creating thrombi to plug up vessel damage, there aren't many left over for normal clotting needs and a patient's clotting time will increase, meaning they bleed for too long. Gums might bleed during daily tooth brushing, or needle sticks for lab work might drip blood for longer than usual. At its worst, a person is pretty much

[90] Arya Mariam Roy, Manojna Konda, Akshay Goel, Appalanaidu Sasapu; Epidemiology and Factors Affecting Mortality of Hospitalized Patients with Disseminated Intravascular Coagulation in the United States. *Blood* 2019; 134 (Supplement_1): 2404. doi: https://doi.org/10.1182/blood-2019-132071

bleeding all over the place for no reason. You might see large pools of blood collecting under their skin, making reddish-purple patches all over their body. For anyone who has ever lived as a human, it should be pretty obvious why this is a very, very bad thing.

Now this is clearly a worst-case scenario, but these complications are why blood pressure has to be monitored so closely in pregnancy. We want to prevent preeclampsia from turning into eclampsia, and we want to avoid HELLP and DIC like the plague.

For simple cases of gestational hypertension, blood pressure can be closely monitored and managed with medications. Many women reading this book will experience high blood pressure during pregnancy, and in most cases go on to deliver very healthy, happy babies after taking routine medications.

If preeclampsia is diagnosed in the third trimester, which it usually is, the goal is monitoring the pregnancy until the fetus reaches a point of viability. Then doctors will induce labor as soon as it's safe. If seizures start, eclampsia in the third trimester is typically treated with an emergency c-section. Rule of thumb is this: deliver the baby and the hypertension goes away.

However, if hypertension progresses to severe pre-eclampsia or eclampsia before the 24-week mark, it's usually serious. Abortion may be suggested depending on the patient's specific symptoms and depending on how early in the pregnancy it is. That's because the sooner pre-eclampsia starts causing organ damage, the more likely it is to have serious or life-threatening effects later on. As for eclampsia, the only definitive care is to remove the baby and placenta from the body by delivery, which can be induced early if the baby is old enough, or done as an abortion if the fetus is not yet viable. By taking swift action, strokes, coma and brain damage can be avoided on the maternal side. However, if eclampsia is allowed to continue, it can lead to intrauterine growth restriction[91] or fetal demise on the fetus side and placental abruption, HELLP, DIC, stroke, renal failure, postpartum hemorrhage, and death on the maternal side.

Remember: With hypertension, it's all about timing and severity. While this is mostly a non-issue, it may be a case for abortion if it's both symptomatic and early in the pregnancy.

Premature rupture of membranes

When a person gives birth, the amniotic sac ruptures and leaks fluid. This is what parents mean when they shout, "my water broke!!", while waddling to the car with a hospital bag. When this happens before 24 weeks, it's considered to be before fetal viability, and it's not the best situation for either baby or mom. However, this topic is not as black and white as other complications because what's considered "pretty bad" is entirely subjective and it's difficult to get a clear picture of what the stats are surrounding premature membrane ruptures.

One French paper acknowledged just that, and sought to quantify outcomes in preterm membrane rupture cases. They reviewed 1,435 cases and found that infants survived until discharge only 14.1% of the time if the membranes ruptured at 22 weeks, 39.5% survived until discharge if rupture occurred at 23 weeks, 66.8% at 24 weeks, and 75.8% at 25 weeks.[92] Chances of survival were much higher at both 24 and 25 weeks which is in line with 24 weeks being considered a common

---

[91] Dacaj, R., Izetbegovic, S., Stojkanovic, G., & Dreshaj, S. (2016). Elevated Liver Enzymes in Cases of Preeclampsia and Intrauterine Growth Restriction. *Medical archives (Sarajevo, Bosnia and Herzegovina)*, *70*(1), 44–47. https://doi.org/10.5455/medarh.2016.70.44-47

[92] Lorthe, E., Torchin, H., Delorme, P., Ancel, P. Y., Marchand-Martin, L., Foix-L'Hélias, L., Benhammou, V., Gire, C., d'Ercole, C., Winer, N., Sentilhes, L., Subtil, D., Goffinet, F., & Kayem, G. (2018). Preterm premature rupture of membranes at 22-25 weeks' gestation: perinatal and 2-year outcomes within a national population-based study (EPIPAGE-2). *American journal of obstetrics and gynecology*, *219*(3), 298.e1–298.e14. https://doi.org/10.1016/j.ajog.2018.05.029

marker of viability. Including all surviving infants, less than half made it to their second birthday without cerebral palsy.

The paper also showed that the majority of deliveries happened within a week of membrane rupture.

There is not one right answer for how to care for a pregnant patient with ruptured membranes at 23 weeks. If there are no complications and the patient is receptive to recommended medical care, she may be encouraged to allow the pregnancy to develop to a point of increased viability. During this time, a doctor may choose to give corticosteroids to help the baby's lungs develop, antibiotics to prevent infections, and/or medications to prevent labor.

The ethics of premature birth: Ending a pregnancy isn't the only reproductive hot topic. Premature rupture of membranes is more often a question of "to induce or not to induce" than a question of abortion. And then, what happens after delivery? What about a 22 week pregnancy with premature membrane rupture and signs of infection? The baby has not reached a point of viability and has about a 28% chance of survival.

After delivery, should a hospital be required to provide invasive procedures like artificial ventilation in a newborn who is unlikely to survive? Should a family be allowed the choice to mourn, holding their newborn for the limited time they have together?

Bell EF, Hintz SR, Hansen NI, et al. Mortality, In-Hospital Morbidity, Care Practices, and 2-Year Outcomes for Extremely Preterm Infants in the US, 2013-2018. *JAMA.* 2022;327(3):248–263. doi:10.1001/jama.2021.23580

Once a fetus has reached the third trimester, the goal in premature rupture involving a healthy, developmentally normal fetus, would be to delay labor as long as it's considered safe. If a pregnancy gets to 37 weeks, it's likely to be a relatively normal delivery.

However, if an infection develops after rupture, things start to change since this poses the risk of sepsis to both the newborn baby and mom (sepsis is a life-threatening reaction to infection causing system wide dysfunction and organ damage). An embryo or fetus typically needs to be delivered or removed soon after infection is found regardless of fetal viability.

Placental Problems

Placental abruption

Before reading this section, make sure you understand implantation as described in chapter six. How the placenta develops is key to understanding how this brand new, pregnancy-specific organ can go wrong.

Placental abruption is what we call it when the placenta rips off the uterine wall. While we don't always know why this happens, it's more likely in pregnancies to parents over 35 years old, smokers, and habitual drug users. It can also result from blunt trauma (a car accident, physical abuse, etc.) or increased pressure from preeclampsia/eclampsia.

Remember, the placenta is the main source of blood, nutrients and oxygen to the fetus. If this supply is interrupted, fetal demise is possible. As the placenta rips off the uterine wall, bleeding will occur. If this happens near the edges of the placenta, some blood may leak out of the vagina, sending the message that something has gone wrong. However, if it occurs in the center of the placenta, a pocket of blood will form internally without any visible bleeding. Either way, the uterus will tense up to prevent further blood loss and the mother will feel pain in her abdomen or pelvis.

A minor bleed may be no cause for concern and can go totally unnoticed until delivery. In this case, if there aren't any changes in the health of the parent or fetus, the pregnancy can be monitored closely and may be able to progress normally.

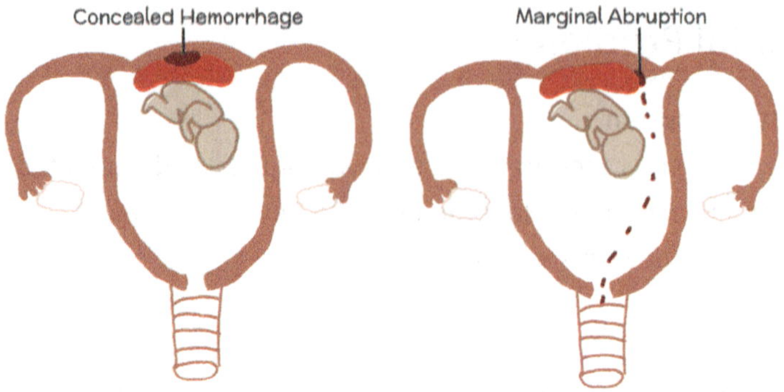

However, a large tear can quickly lead to dangerous blood loss, hypovolemic shock (caused by blood loss), renal failure, DIC (review the eclampsia section if you forgot what this terrible syndrome is), and Sheehan syndrome (damage to the pituitary gland from blood loss). If enough blood is not being delivered to the fetus, it will not survive.

If placental abruption is causing complications on the maternal or fetal side, delivery via c-section is the only option to prevent death due to blood loss. If this happens before the point of fetal viability, an emergency c-section may become an abortion if it results in fetal loss.

Genetic and developmental complications

Discussing maternal complications like gestational trophoblastic neoplasm and eclampsia is a difficult, complicated topic. Compare that to discussing fetal complications and I'll take the maternal side of the conversation any day. This section, while short, may be emotionally taxing to read. I know it was draining to write.

The question of life and the quality of that life become an ethical rather than a scientific question almost immediately when it comes to genetic issues, birth defects, and disability. While I've put some thought-provoking questions below, I'm going to do my best to stay away from ethical statements. You can refer to the chapter on development for more information on when life may, or may not, truly begin, but at the end of the day, that's a call everyone needs to make on their own. As far as quality of life, I don't feel this book is the appropriate place to argue for, or against, the life of any child. What I will do is suggest that if you have strong feelings on the appropriateness of terminating a pregnancy with a genetic condition, review the chapter on IVF and ask yourself if you have the same moral qualms with Preimplantation Genetic Testing as you do with abortion for the same reasons. Why or why not?

Screening: When are fetal abnormalities and genetic defects diagnosed?

One of the many routine tests done during pregnancy is the ultrasound. During this procedure, a technician will squirt an unnecessarily cold goop all over the abdomen and then rub a transducer against the skin. Sound waves bounce off the structures inside the pelvis to create an image of the uterus and embryo/fetus. Sometimes, abnormalities will be visible between 10-14 weeks that indicate neural tube defects and/or other genetic disorders like trisomy 12, 18, and 21. If any abnormalities are detected, additional blood tests, amniocentesis and/or chorionic villus sampling can be done to confirm diagnosis.

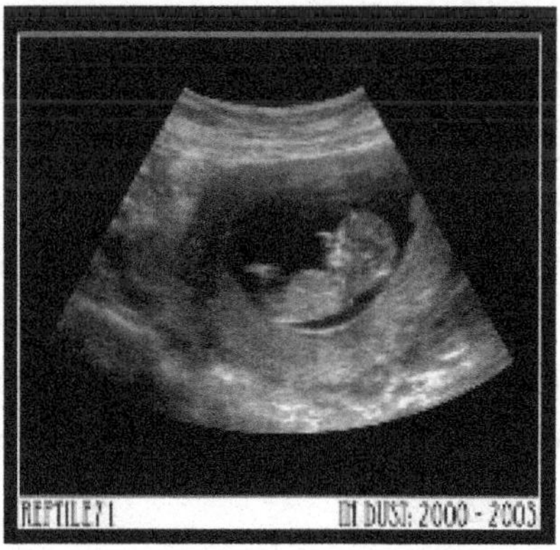

Wikimedia commons image:
https://commons.wikimedia.org/wiki/File:Indust.jpg

In updated guidelines from the American College of Medical Genetics and Genomics, maternal serum alpha-fetoprotein (MSAFP) is suggested as a routine maternal blood test between 16-18 weeks of pregnancy.[93] This lab looks for elevated alpha-fetoprotein which can diagnose neural tube defects 75%-95% of the time. Additionally, another maternal blood test called a quad screen (including MSAFP, hCG, uE3, and INH-A levels) can help detect trisomies 13, 18, and 21.

For women over 35 years old, or pregnancies that have an abnormal ultrasound, an amniocentesis or chorionic villus sampling (CVS) may be done to review any abnormalities. In an amniocentesis, a very long (but very thin) needle is inserted into the abdomen, through the uterine wall, and into the amniotic sac where it draws out a small amount of amniotic fluid. The fluid will have enough fetal DNA to test for genetic abnormalities including trisomies or known genetic disorders. Unlike serum lab tests that only require a quick blood draw from mom, amniocentesis is invasive and comes with a 0.6% chance of miscarriage within two weeks after the procedure.[94] It's also not recommended before 15 weeks of pregnancy which presents an issue for parents who discover a genetic defect at 16+ weeks pregnant that they're unwilling or unable to deal with since this falls outside of 6, 10, and 12 week abortion bans.

If there is a high risk factor for genetic defects, parents can opt for chorionic villus sampling earlier than amniocentesis, between 10-12 weeks of pregnancy, which would give them more time to make decisions. Again, a long thin needle is inserted into the uterus but a small sample is taken from the placenta instead of the amniotic fluid. This procedure comes with the same very small risk of miscarriage.

---

[93] Driscoll, D., the Professional Practice and Guidelines Committee. Second trimester maternal serum screening for fetal open neural tube defects and aneuploidy. *Genet Med* 6, 540–541 (2004). https://doi.org/10.1097/00125817-200411000-00013

[94] *Virtual Mentor.* 2008;10(5):304-306. doi: 10.1001/virtualmentor.2008.10.5.cprl1-0805.

Some disorders doctors screen for:
While I only chose to include neural tube defects and chromosomal count abnormalities in this chapter, there are hundreds of genetic conditions a person may want to test for including Fragile X, cystic fibrosis, beta thalassemia, and more.

Neural tube defects

Finding stats on pregnancies in the United States that were terminated specifically due to neural tube defects was a difficult task. I did, however, come across a huge compilation of data from England and Wales spanning from 2007-2017 that tracks terminations for three neural tube defects: anencephaly (missing parts of the brain and/or skull), encephalocele (when the brain bulges into a bubble protruding from the skull), and spina bifida (when part of the spinal cord sticks out of the body),[95] as well as international studies on neural tube defects and termination of pregnancy due to fetal anomaly (TOPFA).

The development of these conditions happens between day 24-26 after fertilization when the neural tube is closing (review chapter six as a reminder). If the tube fails to close, the fetus will have one of these three defects depending on where the closure failure happens: the anterior neuropore results in anencephaly, near the top is encephalocele, and the middle or caudal end is spina bifida.

---

[95] Allen, R, James, A, Sankaran, S. Trends in termination of pregnancy for neural tube defects in England and Wales from 2007 to 2017: observational prospective study. *Prenat Diagn*. 2021; 41(13): 1624- 1633. https://doi.org/10.1002/pd.6060

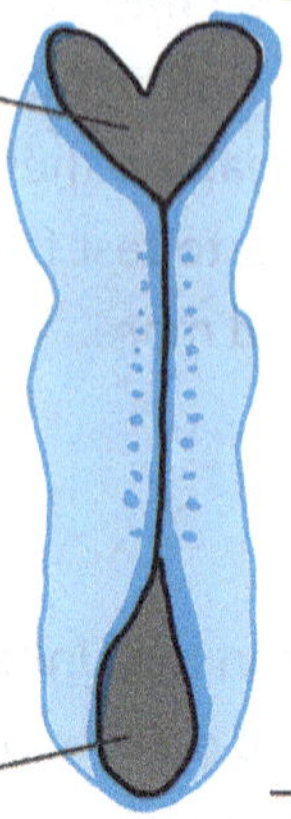

Anencephaly: In anencephaly, the portion of the brain responsible for higher level thought and critical thinking is most commonly missing, meaning these babies will have minimal developmental ability if they survive into childhood. In some cases, the *majority* of brain tissue will fail to develop. In an analysis of data from around the world, women who live in countries with access to elective abortion procedures chose to end a pregnancy with anencephaly 90.6% of the time.[96]

- Note, anencephaly is not the same as microcephaly (micro = "small, "cephaly" = related to the head). While anencephaly is a neural tube defect, having a small head and/or brain is typically caused by gene mutations or, more recently, Zika virus. Unfortunately, microcephaly can go unnoticed on ultrasound until the second or third trimesters, if it's ever noticed at all pre-birth. This means that families may not find out until late in a pregnancy, when abortions are often banned, that a fetus has this problem.

[96] Blencowe, H., Kancherla, V., Moorthie, S., Darlison, M.W. and Modell, B. (2018), Estimates of global and regional prevalence of neural tube defects for 2015: a systematic analysis. Ann. N.Y. Acad. Sci., 1414: 31-46. https://doi.org/10.1111/nyas.13548

Encephalocele: In this case, the brain bulges from the skull. If it's only a small bit being pushed out into the face or nose, it may go undetected and cause little to no issue for the child. However, if the brain bulges from the back of the skull, it's extremely likely that the baby will have neurological deficits. While surgery can be done to put the brain back where it belongs, it cannot reverse any neurological damage. Symptoms can include paralysis, seizures, developmental/intellectual delays, and vision problems. 61.7% of women with access to elective abortions chose not to have babies who were diagnosed with encephalocele.

When poverty and reproductive rights collide: Consuming 300-400 mcg of folic acid a day by taking prenatal vitamins can prevent neural tube defects. By week 6 of pregnancy (4 weeks after conception, 2 weeks after a person's first missed period) the neural tube is already closed. What happens when a person doesn't know to take supplements in time or doesn't have the financial resources to purchase them?

In one paper, researchers found that fewer than 5% of low income mothers took prenatal vitamins before pregnancy. More often, they started after week 4-6 when the neural tube was already closed.

If a person without access to, or knowledge about, prenatal vitamins discovers her baby has no brain, should she be required to maintain the pregnancy and give birth?

Cheng, T. L., Mistry, K. B., Wang, G., Zuckerman, B., & Wang, X. (2018). Folate Nutrition Status in Mothers of the Boston Birth Cohort, Sample of a US Urban Low-Income Population. *American journal of public health*, 108(6), 799–807. https://doi.org/10.2105/AJPH.2018.304355

Spina bifida: This is one of the more complicated diagnoses when it comes to neural tube defects because the effect on a future child is not clear cut. Spina bifida can range from an open myelomeningocele where the spinal cord and meninges are protruding from the back and exposed to the world, to a small gap in between the vertebrae that causes no physical issue. If a myelomeningocele is present, loss of sensation and function below the opening is likely. This can lead to incontinence and paralysis.

Despite having a wide range of severity from asymptomatic to life-limiting, 73.8% of women chose to terminate these pregnancies if possible.

Trisomy and related chromosomal count issues

A normal human has 46 chromosomes in every cell and those 46 chromosomes organize themselves into 23 pairs. One set comes from the maternal parent, and the other from the paternal parent. I didn't delve into meiosis and mitosis (cell division) to avoid getting bogged down in the details, but in short, chromosomal abnormalities are usually a result of a flawed cell division process. When gametes (eggs/oocytes in women and sperm in men) are created, they end up being haploid. That means instead of 23 pairs of chromosomes, they only have 23 chromosomes total. That way, when an egg and sperm meet, there is one copy from mom and one from dad making 46 chromosomes organized into 23 pairs in the new embryo.

The most common cause of trisomies is when eggs are formed and nondisjunction happens. This is exactly what it sounds like. The DNA does not (non-) undergo disjunction (separation of chromosomes). Because of this, one egg will have two copies of a single chromosome from the maternal side, instead of one copy. When it is fertilized by a sperm, there are three copies of that specific chromosome with two from mom and one from dad. We usually only see this happen with Trisomy 21 (Down syndrome), Trisomy 18 (Edward's syndrome) and Trisomy 13 (Patau Syndrome). Down syndrome is the most common of all of these considering newborns with Trisomy 18 and 13 are far less likely to survive.

Another way trisomies happen is when a healthy embryo with a proper amount of DNA is formed. Early in embryo development, as cells divide rapidly, one of the cells has a random mutation and ends up with a trisomy. Because the early cells in an embryo will go on to create the rest of the cells in the body, this means that all cells derived from the mutated one will also have trisomy. This is called mosaicism and can lead to a less severe version of the syndromes listed here due to the fact that some cells in the baby will be typical and others will have three copies of the specific gene.

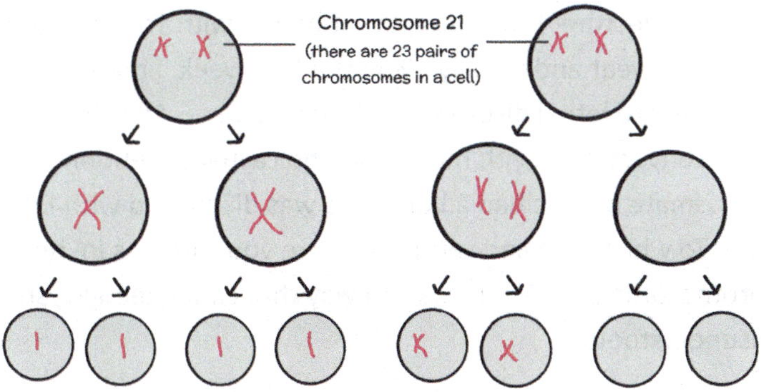

Normal division creates 4 haploid eggs, all with 1 copy of chromosome 21

Nondisjunction creates 2 eggs with 2 copies of chromosome 21 and 2 eggs with none

Mosaicism

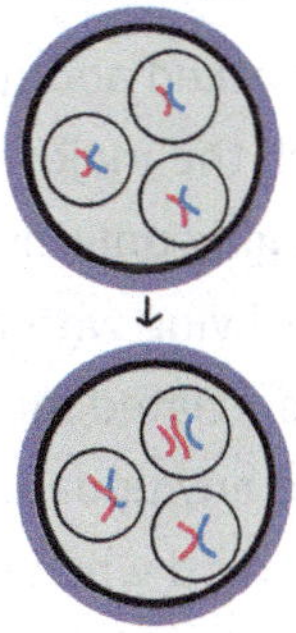

During cell division a mutation in the early embyro creates a cell with trisomy

If trisomy occurs, abnormalities may show up on ultrasound as soon as the first trimester. Blood work including a Quad screen can give a parent more information, but definitive diagnosis is usually done via amniocentesis.

Trisomies with Low Life Expectancy

The likelihood of these babies dying in utero, during birth, or within the first year of life is extremely high. While carrying a fetus with trisomy 13 or 18 does not typically cause harm to the mother during pregnancy, it does take an emotional and mental toll. If someone has the full form of these syndromes (not mosaicism), it's virtually unheard of to have one of these children survive to adulthood. Notice the word "virtually".

In one genetics lecture, I was taught that babies with Trisomy 18 *never* survive the first year and usually die in the first week. I memorized the fact that these are lethal disorders 100% of the time. And then I found myself in a conversation with my friend who casually mentioned that a former classmate of hers had a baby who was diagnosed with Edward's syndrome. To which I replied cautiously, "are you sure? As in, he has an extra chromosome 18?" There was no way that could be right, she must have misunderstood.

But, yes. She was 100 percent sure.

The child was still alive when I asked about them multiple years later. This child will likely never reach the majority of developmental milestones, for example, it's highly unlikely they will ever be capable of forming words.[97] The child was living with full time, around the clock care and was a well-loved, appreciated member of their small little family at the time (I don't have any updates since). Likely, their story is one of the many case studies I read when writing this chapter since we still have so few examples of older children living with these conditions. These scattered cases allow physicians to see what happens when the rare trisomy 13 and 18 patients live into their teenage years.

While I'm not making a statement on quality of life, and would encourage anyone seeking more information to discuss life with families who are living with this disorder, the fact remains, the vast majority of these children will still not survive and it's very important that families with these pregnancies are realistic about potential outcomes.

Trisomy 13 - Patau Syndrome - Having a third copy of chromosome 13 is the most severe of the trisomies. If a pregnancy with Patau syndrome is successfully carried to term (depending on the source, around 50% end

---

[97] Barbara Braddock, Jena McDaniel, Sara Spragge, Filip Loncke, Stephen R. Braddock & John C. Carey (2012) Communication Ability in Persons with Trisomy 18 and Trisomy 13, Augmentative and Alternative Communication, 28:4, 266-277, DOI: 10.3109/07434618.2012.706637

in spontaneous abortion or stillbirth[98]), newborns may have neural tube defects, congenital heart issues, extra fingers and toes, a cleft lip, hearing loss, seizures, missing or underdeveloped eyes, and severe learning/developmental disabilities. Out of live births, less than 10% will survive 5 years.[99]

Trisomy 18 - Edwards Syndrome - In Trisomy 18, the likelihood of stillbirth or spontaneous abortion is noticeably higher at over 70%, but the babies that result from live births are slightly more likely to survive to year five (about 12%). These newborns may have congenital heart defects, neural tube defects, cleft lips and scoliosis. Every child born with this condition will have life-altering developmental delays that prevent them from achieving any level of independence.

Most common Trisomy: Trisomy 21 - Down Syndrome - It's likely that you've met someone or know of a relative or friend-of-a-friend who has Down Syndrome. As children and adults, people with trisomy 21 will typically have a lower-than-average IQ, congenital heart defects, problems with their GI tract, and developmental delays. One of the genes on chromosome 21 happens to code for proteins implicated in the onset of Alzheimer's which explains why many patients with Down Syndrome will be diagnosed with the early onset variation of the disease. The chance of fetal demise in utero or during birth is

---

[98]Morris, J. K., & Savva, G. M. (2008). The risk of fetal loss following a prenatal diagnosis of trisomy 13 or trisomy 18. *American journal of medical genetics. Part A, 146A*(7), 827–832. https://doi.org/10.1002/ajmg.a.32220

[99]Meyer, R. E., Liu, G., Gilboa, S. M., Ethen, M. K., Aylsworth, A. S., Powell, C. M., Flood, T. J., Mai, C. T., Wang, Y., Canfield, M. A., & National Birth Defects Prevention Network (2016). Survival of children with trisomy 13 and trisomy 18: A multi-state population-based study. *American journal of medical genetics. Part A, 170A*(4), 825–837. https://doi.org/10.1002/ajmg.a.37495

somewhere between 10%-12%,[100] [101] but when carried to term, the majority of these babies will survive the first year of life and adults with this disorder can live well into their 60s.

With Trisomy 21, survival is much more likely than other trisomies, and some people with this disorder will have only mild cognitive impairment. Living independently will still be difficult in most cases and additional resources are needed throughout these kid's educational careers. However, people with Down syndrome are fully capable of expressing emotion, loving their family and friends, engaging in conversation, and being physically independent (walking, feeding, sleeping, etc.) in most cases and in some cases of mosaicism may be virtually unaffected.

Single gene defects

The number of disorders we can narrow down to a single mutated or defective gene reaches well into the hundreds. If I listed all of them here, I might as well write a genetics textbook and I'm not going to do that since there's almost nothing I can imagine that sounds more tedious. So instead, I'll say this – single gene disorders can be as equally, or more, devastating than trisomies or neural tube defects. In some cases, parents have had to witness the decline, disability, and death of loved ones with heritable conditions only to see the same disorder pop up during prenatal genetic testing. As much as society might like to issue a moral ruling on babies with genetic disorders and their right to live or not, it's impossible to truly understand the reality of a parent grappling with this decision.

---

[100]Won, R. H., Currier, R. J., Lorey, F., & Towner, D. R. (2005). The timing of demise in fetuses with trisomy 21 and trisomy 18. *Prenatal diagnosis*, *25*(7), 608–611. https://doi.org/10.1002/pd.1243

[101] Springer, S., Karner, E., Worda, C., Grabner, M. M., Seidl-Mlczoch, E., Laccone, F., Neesen, J., Scharrer, A., & Ulm, B. (2022). Outcome after Prenatal Diagnosis of Trisomy 13, 18, and 21 in Fetuses with Congenital Heart Disease. *Life (Basel, Switzerland)*, *12*(8), 1223. https://doi.org/10.3390/life12081223

Genetic counseling can help future parents determine the likelihood of having a child with a certain trait or gene, but it's impossible to prevent passing on some conditions unless the family uses donor eggs or sperm. CNY Fertility, a major fertility treatment company, reported that in 2010 the average cost of IVF using an egg donor in the US was $38,000, an unattainable sum for so many families.[102] Because of cost restrictions, many families may choose to go ahead with a natural pregnancy and then do chorionic villus sampling and extra screening in the first trimester to help ensure the baby is developing normally.

If genetic disorders show up during screening, parents may choose to terminate that pregnancy rather than bring a life into this world that will suffer from a disorder that they believe will only lead to sadness and loss. Should this be a regulated decision or should it be the choice of the parents and their ability to handle the additional needs of a child with a genetic abnormality?

---

[102] CNY Fertility. (2021, December 2). *Donor Egg Cost & financing: The average cost of donor egg IVF in USA*. CNY Fertility. https://www.cnyfertility.com/donor-egg-cost/#costs-of-infertility-treatment-results-from-an-18-month-prospective-cohort-study

Chapter 10

Consent and violation

While I've made light of so many aspects of female reproduction in this book, the following chapter is written without levity. Every sentence in this chapter may trigger those who have suffered sexual trauma. Below you'll find a list of subtopics with page numbers if you would like to read a specific bit of information without going through the rest.

I would also like to make one point as clear as possible to all readers before we go any further. **Penetrative vaginal sex involves the same physical mechanics and occurs within the same ovarian and menstrual cycles both if it's consensual and if it's not.** There is no difference from a biological perspective related to ovulation, fertilization and pregnancy. Women cannot clamp down their vaginal walls to prevent a penis from entering. The presence of natural lubrication does not mean a woman "wants it". Hormonal cycles are not interrupted by unwanted penetration any more than wanted penetration. Pregnancy is no less likely in the case of sexual assault and implying a woman is less likely to get pregnant if she "doesn't want to" is not only biologically inaccurate, but wildly hurtful to survivors.

Please take note of the full stops after each one of those sentences. If anything written above goes against your current beliefs, I beg you to read on with an open mind and review the academic articles I've included as references in the paragraphs below. I've done my best to include no information from popular news sources and instead cite the Department of Justice, or scholarly publications to avoid any arguments of the mainstream media being biased. The exception to this rule is when I reference examples from pop culture or politics, although these aren't used as much to make a point as they are to demonstrate when you might see these topics pop up in the real world. Additionally, make sure you have a firm understanding of the anatomy and physiology in the first few chapters of this book to truly understand the processes below.

The virginity exam

While we'd all like to think "the virginity test" is an outdated relic of the past, we saw how untrue that was when in 2019, rapper T.I. claimed he had his 18-year-old daughter go for hymen checks every year to ensure her virginity.[103] I'm tempted to dismiss this as a bizarre one-off occurrence in modern America, but a popularly cited survey in 2016 says otherwise. It turns out 10% of US Obstetrician–Gynecologists (OBGYNs) had been asked about virginity testing or hymen restoration in the 12 months preceding the survey. 3.5% of surveyed physicians admitted to

---

[103] Ferré-sadurní, L. (2019, December 3). *After the rapper T.I.'s remarks, N.Y. may ban "virginity tests."* The New York Times. https://www.nytimes.com/2019/12/03/nyregion/virginity-test-ti-ny-law.html

performing virginity tests on request.[104] If you missed that, read it again. There are doctors in the United States, in this decade, who are checking a woman's virginity with a physical exam.

The whole concept is mind-boggling considering hymens have a huge amount of natural variation including flower patterns, lumps, bumps, half-crescents, fully intact coverings, and more. A person *can* be born without this little flap of skin partially covering their vaginal opening, but it's very rare at less than .03% of newborns.[105] So, most vaginas *do* come equipped with hymens, but this piece of skin doesn't tear as easily or as frequently as previously thought. Even with penetration, they don't tear every time. The whole idea of a virginity exam proving if someone has been penetrated or not is completely inaccurate.

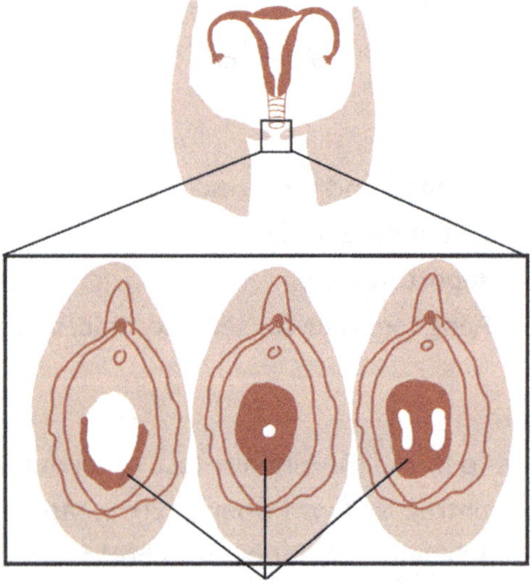

Examples of Hymen Variation

---

[104] Moaddab, A., McCullough, L. B., Chervenak, F. A., Stark, L., Schulkin, J., Dildy, G. A., Raine, S. P., & Shamshirsaz, A. A. (2017). A survey of honor-related practices among US obstetricians and gynecologists. *International journal of gynaecology and obstetrics: the official organ of the International Federation of Gynaecology and Obstetrics, 139*(2), 164–169. https://doi.org/10.1002/ijgo.12294

[105] Jenny C, Kuhns ML, Arakawa F. Hymens in newborn female infants. Pediatrics. 1987 Sep;80(3):399-400. PMID: 3627892.

If you've ever watched a historical drama, you've probably witnessed the popular wedding night scene play out where two people get married, consummate their marriage, and then have family members or servants confirm the successful night with an inspection of the bedsheets for blood. In real life, it turns out that seeing blood on the bed sheets is a terrible way to confirm someone's loss of virginity. What multiple studies show is that in the case of penetration, the hymen often does *not* tear, and the genitalia remains fully intact,[106] especially in younger women. Sadly, a lot of the data we have comes from sexual abuse victims in the pediatric community and is a poignant reminder of why hymen checks should never be used to refute a sexual abuse claim. Even if a hymen is intact, vaginal penetration may have happened. And it may have happened forcefully, without consent.

Why am I spending so much time talking about these checks? In more religious or conservative communities, they are still performed as a confirmation of purity before and after marriage (Does the woman appear to be intact before the wedding night during a visual exam? Was there blood after the wedding night confirming consummation of the marriage?). Women are not always given the choice to deny these checks and they may be done by untrained acquaintances rather than medical professionals. When a hymen exam also includes its cousin, "the two-finger check", the person doing it not only visually examines the hymen, but inserts two fingers into the vagina. In this case, it's not just embarrassment that's at stake, but being penetrated by another person's fingers. In Pakistan, for example, the two-finger test was regularly used up until 2021 to determine if a woman's claim of rape was legitimate or not.

One of the more public abuses of this exam happened during Egyptian protests in 2011 when soldiers did virginity exams to determine the

---

[106] Gallion, H. R., Milam, L. J., & Littrell, L. L. (2016). Genital Findings in Cases of Child Sexual Abuse: Genital vs Vaginal Penetration. *Journal of pediatric and adolescent gynecology*, *29*(6), 604–611. https://doi.org/10.1016/j.jpag.2016.05.001

purity of detained protestors.[107] To the Egyptian government's credit, the practice was acknowledged by the military and outlawed within a year of it going public. But it's not just faraway lands that have used this entirely flawed exam. For example, British immigration officers in the 1970s prescribed these checks to ensure foreign fiancées of British nationals were not previously wed. The thinking at the time was that a foreign woman might try to sneak into Britain as a spouse even if she was already married in her own country so it was better to check first. Apparently, when free love was all the rage in the United States, premarital sex was still unheard of across the pond. Up to 80 women were subjected to vaginal exams during that time.[108] As of 2023, the virginity check has been formally banned in the UK, Bangladesh, Pakistan and India. There are no laws regarding the practice in the United States.

How do we prove "rape"?

Now, we know the hymen will not always tear from penetrative sex. Someone being intact is not necessarily a way to prove, or disprove, penetration. Then how do we prove sex, especially of the nonconsensual variety? And why is proof so important?

In the United States, a person may choose to report a rape to the local police department and/or go to a hospital and ask for a Sexual Assault Evidence Kit (rape kit). This is a forensic exam, designed for evidence gathering. However, by completing a rape kit, a person does not have to formally report their attacker. Collecting evidence simply provides them the option of using it to pursue charges later.

---

[107] Amnesty International. (2021, June 23). *Egypt: Military pledges to stop forced "virginity tests."* Amnesty International. https://www.amnesty.org/en/latest/press-release/2011/06/egypt-military-pledges-stop-forced-virginity-tests/

[108] Travis, A. (2011, May 8). *Virginity tests for immigrants "reflected dark age prejudices" of 1970s Britain*. The Guardian. https://www.theguardian.com/uk/2011/may/08/virginity-tests-immigrants-prejudices-britain

Unfortunately, not all samples are tested and the time frame for storage varies greatly by region. Therefore, it's important for a survivor to understand the statute of limitations in their region and how long their kit will be saved for.

> *Protecting kits:* Rape kits and their disposal were the driving factor behind the Sexual Assault Survivors' Rights Act passed with bipartisan support in 2016 after being introduced by Mimi Walters (Republican) and Zoe Lofgren (Democrat).
> This act protects the right to:
> 1. Free access to a sexual assault kit
> 2. Storage of a kit until the statute of limitations runs out for a person to report or charge their attacker with sexual assault
> 3. Information regarding the to the results, location, and status of a kit
>
> Refer to 18 U.S. Code § 3772 for the full text

Common belief is that these kits should be done within 72 hours of the event, preferably before a person showers, goes to the bathroom, or changes their clothing. Although the right to a kit is now protected by the Sexual Assault Survivors' Rights Act, its use may be discouraged by medical professionals who have been trained on a strict 72 hours cutoff. Sgt. Joanne Archambault, retired from the San Diego Police Department, wrote a wonderful piece in 2007 on why timing is not as important as we think, and evidence collection may be inadequate in many cases because medical professionals prioritize medical treatment over evidence.[109]

What do I mean by collection being inadequate? If a woman requests a rape kit after 96 hours, she might be verbally discouraged due to the futility of her request. However, bodily fluids on a pair of underwear or a couch cushion may last well beyond 96 hours. As for semen in a vagina? We're not really sure how long that can last but some reports have argued it can be found weeks after the act. The 72-hour rule was most likely made in relation to medical procedures (treating lesions caused by violent assault, preventing STIs, and providing emergency contraceptives) and isn't necessarily relevant to evidence collection.

---

[109]Archambault, J., Time Limits for Conducting a Forensic Examination: Can Biological Evidence be Recovered 24, 36, 48, 72, 84 or 96 Hours Following a Sexual Assault?, Sexual Assault Report, Civic Research Institute Inc., Kingston, NJ, Volume 10, Number 3, January/February 2007, p 33-47

Apparently, sexual assault kits shouldn't be argued about or regulated by doctors at all. They should be within the realm of forensic specialists and merely carried out by physicians and nurses.

What does a "rape kit" include?

During an ideal examination, a healthcare professional trained in sexual assault treatment (a Sexual Assault Nurse Examiner/SANE, Sexual Assault Forensic Examiner/SAFE, or Sexual Assault Examiners/SAE)[110] will start by asking the patient a series of questions including a request to describe the physical encounter in detail and explain any other sexual acts that occurred in the previous days both consensual and not. The goal of these questions is to determine if there will be other DNA from consensual activity present and decide if additional areas need to be checked for evidence. For example, if a woman had consensual sex with her husband the night before her assault, and nonconsensual penetrative sex several hours before the exam, it's helpful to note that multiple DNA samples may show up on vaginal swabs. Additionally, if a person's attacker ejaculated on an area of the body other than inside the vagina, that area should be swabbed for DNA collection as well.

Every step from taking a patient's history onwards should be described before proceeding and a patient is given the ability to decline any part of the exam at any time. For the physical portion, a medical provider may use a swab to collect fluids from the vagina and cervix during an internal exam. This swab can be sent to a forensic lab for DNA testing. The exam itself helps a provider determine if any physical trauma is present on the genitalia both for evidence and treatment. For example, bruises and lacerations will be logged, while any actively bleeding wounds may need to be stitched as well. Any hairs or other pieces of evidence found on the body will be collected from a paper placed on the examination table and stored in a plastic bag. Clothes worn during/after the attack should

---

[110] RAINN. (n.d.). *What is a sexual assault forensic exam?*. RAINN. https://www.rainn.org/articles/rape-kit

be collected as well. If there was the possibility a person was drugged before the attack, blood or urine may be taken for a toxicology workup.

Testing: Many STI tests will not show a positive result until multiple days after exposure. However, most sexual assault victims do not return for follow up care, so the following tests are offered during the physical exam as per CDC guidelines:[111]

- NAATs (nucleic acid amplification test using a vaginal swab) for *Chlamydia trachomatis* and *N. gonorrhoeae*
- NAAT testing for *Trichomonas vaginalis*
- Vaginal pH and testing of vaginal secretions for evidence of bacterial vaginosis and candidiasis (yeast infection)
- Serum sample for HIV, HBV, and syphilis infection

Treatment: Because follow-up appointments are poorly attended, antibiotics are suggested on a routine basis for all rape survivors and include ceftriaxone, doxycycline, and metronidazole. These can treat common STIs including chlamydia and gonorrhea.

If an attacker is known or suspected to have HIV/AIDs, treatment with PEP (post-exposure prophylaxis) is advised within 72 hours of the attack including a 28-day supply of tenofovir, emtricitabine, and either dolutegravir or raltegravir. These drugs drastically reduce the risk of getting HIV after exposure.

Once the exam is over, patients can choose if they report the assault to authorities or not. In the case of children and minors, medical providers may be required by law to report. In most cases, adult patients are in control of if they contact police or not. However, a rape is not "proven" by forensic evidence alone in the United States; it's considered a legal matter. Until an attacker is formally charged with rape and proven guilty in court, any accusations remain just that in a legal sense – accusations.

---

[111] *Updated Guidelines for Antiretroviral Postexposure Prophylaxis after Sexual, Injection-Drug Use, or Other Nonoccupational Exposure to HIV – United States, 2016.* MMWR Morb Mortal Wkly Rep, 2016. 65(17): p. 458.

Why would someone wait (or decline) to report sexual assault?
I don't think there's any answer I could write here that would cover the myriad reasons rape goes unreported. What I can do is show you that not only does it sometimes go unreported, it *usually* does. While the #MeToo movement in the United States has encouraged women to speak up about sexual violence, it's also drawn criticism from more conservative sources that nearly anything can be considered sexual assault. Instead of getting lost in the weeds over the believability of women in general and the difference between harassment and assault, I'm going to attempt to discuss only cases of penetrative rape. I encourage any reader to use these facts to deepen your understanding of the prevalence and reality of nonconsensual sex.

According to a report published by the U.S. Bureau of Justice, out of 131,950 completed rapes between 1992 and 2000, 63% were not reported. "Completed rapes" as defined in this report exclude attempted rape and sexual assault. Of those unreported rapes, 83% went untreated, meaning the victim never sought medical care.

That's well over half of completed rapes that never make their way to law enforcement and even more are never treated by a medical provider.

What the report found is that one of the biggest factors in lodging a report is the relationship of the victim to the attacker, "The closer the relationship between the female victim and the offender, the greater the likelihood that the police would not be told about the rape or sexual assault." This little detail is extremely important considering 76% of rapes are perpetrated by a person known to the victim.[112]

---

[112]Jones, J. S., Wynn, B. N., Kroeze, B., Dunnuck, C., & Rossman, L. (2004). Comparison of sexual assaults by strangers versus known assailants in a community-based population. *The American journal of emergency medicine, 22*(6), 454–459. https://doi.org/10.1016/j.ajem.2004.07.020

By far, the majority of rapes are committed by a person known to the survivor. And the biggest deterrent of a person reporting an attack is knowing the survivor. Do you see the connection?

Additionally, in a study comparing victim blaming related to various factors, it was found that if the perpetrator of a rape is an acquaintance, the likelihood that the victim will be blamed for the assault is higher. So, not only are these incidents less likely to be reported, but they have a higher likelihood of being disputed by friends, family, and law enforcement.

Now let's tackle the belief that nonconsensual sex is less harmful if it's committed by an acquaintance. In fact, anogenital injuries in both known and unknown attacker scenarios were found to be comparable (although unknown assailants did tend to cause more injury to other parts of the body).

Aside from the matter of closeness to the perpetrator, another factor cited in failing to report was "fear of reprisal". Stop to consider the fact that 67% of female sexual assault victims are under the age of 18[113] and one of every seven assaults recorded involved children under the age of six. Imagine being a five-year-old victim. How could you *not* be afraid of getting in trouble if you told an adult? Going back to earlier chapters, the onset of puberty typically happens after 8 years old and pregnancy can occur in any uterus that's had its first period.

Think that doesn't have real world consequences? A 10-year-old child in Ohio was reported to be pregnant after Child Protective Services was called to check on her. The man who caused her to become pregnant

---

[113] Bureau of Justice Statistics . (2000). (rep.). *Sexual Assault of Young Children as Reported to Law Enforcement: Victim, Incident, and Offender Characteristics*. Retrieved July 6, 2023, from https://bjs.ojp.gov/library/publications/sexual-assault-young-children-reported-law-enforcement-victim-incident-and.

was a known acquaintance. Shortly after, the Wall Street Journal published an op-ed with the title, "An abortion story too good to confirm".[114] Reporter Tucker Carlson claimed on Fox news that the story was "not true,"[115] and Ohio Attorney General, Dave Yost said there was no evidence of the child existing, to which Ohio Congressman, Jim Jordan tweeted, "another lie."[116]

The child (who was claimed not to exist on a public stage) was denied an abortion in Ohio due to a ban on abortion after a fetal heartbeat was detected. As we learned in the chapter on conception and pregnancy, fetal heartbeats around six weeks are a result of some faint electrical pulses rather than a true heartbeat caused by heart valves opening and closing, but since there were electrical impulses found, it fell within the legal definition of "heartbeat" and she had to travel across state borders to terminate the pregnancy. In the end, it turns out that no amount of victim blaming could change the facts – Gerson Fuentes was matched by DNA evidence from the tissue removed during the abortion and later confessed to raping her on at least two occasions.[117]

While that story illustrates one specific instance, sexual assault is not a singular picture. No two attacks are the same, no two women are the same. The emotional and physical fallout from being violated will look different in everyone.

---

[114] The Wall Street Journal. (2022, July 13). *Opinion | an abortion story too good to confirm*. The Wall Street Journal. https://www.wsj.com/articles/an-abortion-story-too-good-to-confirm-joe-biden-ten-year-old-girl-indiana-ohio-caitlin-bernard-11657648618?redirect=amp

[115] As of the writing of this book, the original news clip can still be found on Twitter at https://twitter.com/Acyn/status/1547330176022978562

[116] As of the writing of this book, the original Tweet can still be found as a screenshot here: https://twitter.com/KFILE/status/1547316940108079111/photo/1

[117] Cook, T., Bruner, B., Trombly, M., & Eom, D. (2022, July 26). *Ohio man charged in rape of 10-year-old that led to Indiana abortion*. The Indianapolis Star. https://www.indystar.com/story/news/2022/07/13/ohio-man-charged-rape-10-year-old-led-indiana-abortion/10048529002/

Where consent, abortion, and contraceptives collide

Let's use a theoretical example of a middle-aged woman who is attacked violently by a stranger, rather than the previous example of a young child being abused by an acquaintance. In this case, fear of reprisal and knowing the attacker are no longer as important. However, there are still factors including religious norms (being considered impure after sex, even if nonconsensual), societal norms (being considered "slutty" or having "asked for it"), and feelings of shame that are a devastating, but normal, part of assault. She doesn't have any open wounds so opts to heal her bruises at home. She doesn't report the rape, but she does pick up the morning after pill at her local pharmacy.

Question for thought: If you typically don't support the use of emergency contraceptives, should a person who seeks medical care within 72 hours of sexual assault be offered the morning after pill as an exception?

Assuming she takes Plan B, ovulation will be prevented and she is unlikely to become pregnant. Access to Plan B is still available in all 50 states, so as long as she overcomes the mental, emotional, and physical barriers to post-assault reporting and medical care, pregnancy shouldn't be an issue.

Right?

Well, that's if she hasn't ovulated yet. Let's say she is assaulted on day 16 of her cycle, a day or two after an egg entered her fallopian tube. She still took Plan B, but it did nothing to prevent pregnancy. Around a month after her last period, she's relieved when she has the same nausea, bloating and tender breasts as she always does before her period. Unfortunately, a week later she still hasn't started menstruating. At this point, she takes a home pregnancy test and sees the tell-tale lines. Immediately, she schedules an appointment with her OBGYN who is willing to see her one week later despite average wait times of 30+

days in most offices. It's now 6 weeks after her last period and about 4 weeks since she was violently taken advantage of. An ultrasound shows she's pregnant despite her best efforts to prevent it. Since she is now 6 weeks pregnant, she's also outside the allotted 6-week time period for abortion that's currently active in states like GA, ID, IA, KY, LA, MS, ND, OH, OK, SC, TN, and TX.

What now?

If she lives in Utah, Mississippi, or Wyoming (as of April 2023), she can still have an abortion with a rape exception despite strict abortion laws. Assuming the rape is reported and a copy of that report is made available to medical staff. In North Dakota, she could skip the reporting, but hopefully she does it fast since all abortion is banned after six weeks.

This type of assault doesn't stand alone as a singular legal issue. Instead, it's intertwined with the larger discussion of reproductive rights.

These kinds of tricky conversations are where the issue of abortion becomes much more than "pro-life" vs. "pro-choice". The *choice* to have sex is stolen from a person in the case of rape. The option to prevent pregnancy is removed when a rapist chooses not to use a condom, especially if it's too late for common emergency contraceptive pills to work. In fact, the right to an abortion in the case of rape or incest is something that almost every human rights organization defends loud and clear. Most notably the UN[118] and the UN Committee Against Torture,[119] the African Court on Human and Peoples' Rights including 54

---

[118] Human Rights Committee, *General Comment No. 36 (2018) on Article 6 of the International Covenant on Civil and Political Rights, on the Right to Life*, at 2, para. 8, U.N. Doc. CCPR/C/GC/36 (2018)

[119] CAT Committee, *Concluding Observations: Nicaragua*, para. 16, U.N. Doc. CAT/C/NIC/CO/1 (2009); CAT Committee, *Concluding Observations: Peru*, para. 23, U.N. Doc. CAT/C/PER/CO/4 (2006).

African Union member states,[120] the Council for Europe Commissioner on Human Rights[121] (particularly in reference to Poland's lack of abortion access), and the World Health Organization (WHO).[122] WHO goes so far as to recommend that the term "rape" in relationship to abortion should be based on a woman's complaint, not physical evidence. A recommendation that makes a lot of sense considering the majority go unreported as it is.

And this culmination of medical fact, law, culture, and reality is where we see the true issues of reproductive rights. How do we encourage reporting and discourage victim blaming? How do we discuss the reality and horror of a physical trauma like rape without getting lost in moral sidebars? And how do we protect the women who are being publicly dragged through these debates?

---

[120] African Commission on Human and Peoples' Rights. (2003). (rep.). *PROTOCOL TO THE AFRICAN CHARTER ON HUMAN AND PEOPLES' RIGHTS ON THE RIGHTS OF WOMEN IN AFRICA*. Retrieved July 6, 2023, from https://www.ohchr.org/sites/default/files/Documents/Issues/Women/WG/ProtocolontheRightsofWomen.pdf.

[121] United Nations Human Rights Office of the High Commissioner . (n.d.). (rep.). *Denial of abortion services and the prohibition of torture and cruel, inhuman and degrading treatment* . Retrieved July 7, 2023, from https://www.ohchr.org/sites/default/files/Documents/Issues/Women/WG/AmicusBrazil.pdf.

[122] World Health Organization. Safe abortion: technical and policy guidance for health systems—2nd ed. Geneva 2012. ISBN 978 92 4 154843 4 http://apps.who.int/iris/bitstream/10665/ 70914/1/9789241548434_eng.pdf

Chapter 11

Why Didn't I Know That?

American schools are famously bad at teaching two things: sex ed and geography (calm down, *I'm* American, and *I'm* bad at geography, I'm not judging you). I put this mini-chapter in here so you can rest assured that you're not alone if you were surprised by how Emergency Contraceptives work, or you had no idea how multi-layered the uterus is – like a meaty onion! American sex education is abysmal. And it's not just us, many countries struggle with the question of when, and how, to discuss the "birds and the bees."

Considering the average age for menstruation in the United States is under 12 years old (between 6th and 7th grade), it would stand to reason that menstruation should be discussed sometime before then. After all, "average" does not mean "beginning at." In fact, 26% of students (more than 1 in 4)[123] will already have their periods by the time they reach 11 years old.

With menstruation comes the possibility of pregnancy, and yet, in the majority of American public schools, sex ed isn't taught until after 6th grade. Menstruation and anatomy are typically bundled with sex ed and separated by gender at that time. For example, in my school, the girls were separated from the boys to discuss periods. I have no idea what the boys were taught – how to hide boners? Wet dreams? Putting condoms on bananas? Regardless, it's not surprising that one of my friends once told me her boyfriend, a guy who grew up in the same area as us, had no idea that women were more likely to get pregnant between their periods. He thought it was all some sort of random crap shoot with equal odds throughout the month.

Now consider that 35-47% of teenagers polled in the United States did not have *any* formal sex education on STIs, or birth control until high school.[124] No conversations about appropriate contraceptives, no talk about STIs, no discussions on HIV. This might explain why so many male politicians, pundits, and policy makers have such a nebulous understanding of what happens leading up to pregnancy.

Between 2011-2015, the CDC reported that 60% of sexually active American teens have relied on one of the least effective methods of birth control on the planet – withdrawal.[125] No wonder the United States has one of the highest teen pregnancy rates out of developed countries. These rates go up in a particular region of the country (the South) and

---

[123] Martinez GM. Trends and patterns in menarche in the United States, 1995 through 2013–2017. National Health Statistics Reports; no 146. Hyattsville, MD: National Center for Health Statistics. 2020.
[124] Martinez G, Abma J, Copen C. Educating teenagers about sex in the United States. NCHS data brief, no 44. Hyattsville, MD: National Center for Health Statistics. 2010.
[125] Abma JC, Martinez GM. Sexual activity and contraceptive use among teenagers in the United States, 2011–2015. National health statistics reports; no 104. Hyattsville, MD: National Center for Health Statistics. 2017.

are noticeably lower on the coasts. For example, the number of teen pregnancies per 1,000 girls are highest in the following states, with over 20 pregnancies/1,000 young women each: Mississippi, Arkansas, Louisiana, Oklahoma, Alabama*, Kentucky, Tennessee, West Virginia*, and Texas*.[126] What do these states have in common? With the exception of Alabama, WV, and Texas, none of them are required to stress contraceptive usage in sex education classrooms, and most don't even have to discuss it.[127] The three outliers, Alabama, West Virginia, and Texas do have legislation related to covering contraceptives, but only on a limited basis. Is it possible girls are getting pregnant simply because they didn't learn about prevention?

Why bring this up in a book related to talking about reproductive issues like a doctor? Having a politician say something absurd about a woman's body is all fine and good for social media fodder, but having a patient believe she can get pregnant through vigorous dry humping, or that she can prevent pregnancy with pennyroyal can cause all sorts of medical confusion and in some cases, patient harm. How do you break the cycle of Americans saying stupid stuff about female bodies?

Read this book. Read another book. Look up *medical* data and sources when you're confused. Understand female anatomy before you discuss female bodies. There is no singular conclusion that needs to be made, but the understanding of facts needs to be there.

The remaining question we have is: If *we're* so bad at sex ed, how do other countries handle all of this?

---

[126] *Teen birth rate comparison, 2020*. Teen Birth Rate Comparison, 2020 | Power to Decide. (n.d.). https://powertodecide.org/what-we-do/information/national-state-data/teen-birth-rate

[127] SIECUS. (2022). (rep.). *Sex Ed State Law and Policy Chart*. Retrieved July 7, 2023, from https://siecus.org/wp-content/uploads/2021/09/2022-Sex-Ed-State-Law-and-Policy-Chart.pdf.

Chapter 12

Comparative Reproduction

In terms of sex education, the majority of European countries have compulsory sex education, with the Dutch being famous for their liberal approach to the topic. In the Netherlands, children begin to learn about appropriate and inappropriate touch in school by age four, and around age 11 they understand the ins-and-outs of contraceptives, conception, and sexual abuse.[128] This approach seems to pay off considering that both Dutch and American teens lose their virginity around the same age, but the rate of teen pregnancies remains much lower in the Netherlands. In fact, teen pregnancy rates are lower in all but four EU member states when compared to the United States. Additionally, Dutch teens are far more likely to use contraceptives during their first sexual

---

[128] Katz, A. (2018, July 19). *Sex ed goes global: The Netherlands*. Global Reproductive Health at Duke. https://dukecenterforglobalreproductivehealth.org/2018/07/19/sex-ed-goes-global-the-netherlands/

experience and report positive feelings surrounding their first time more often than their American peers.[129]

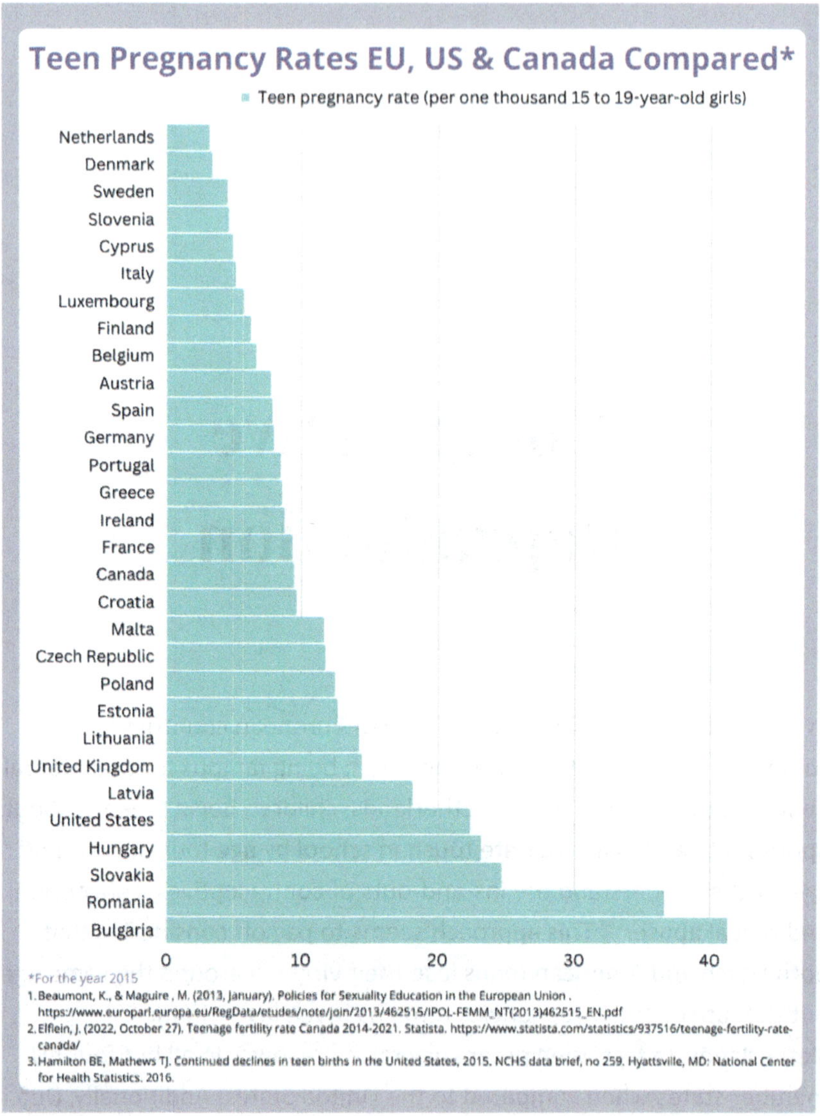

---

[129] Rough, B. J. (2018, August 29). *How the Dutch do sex ed.* The Atlantic. https://www.theatlantic.com/family/archive/2018/08/the-benefits-of-starting-sex-ed-at-age-4/568225/

When it comes to abortion, that's big news since teen pregnancies are often unintended pregnancies and unintended pregnancies are more likely to be terminated.

In the United States, we often think of abortion as a partisan issue. If a person is religious and politically conservative, they will tend to be pro-life. If a person is politically liberal and supportive of LGBTQIA++ rights, they will generally be pro-choice. We Americans tend to use these qualities as a predictive measure for future abortion legislation. Conservative Supreme Court = overturn of Roe V. Wade. A move towards Christian values means a move towards limited reproductive freedom. However, the more I looked at trends in other countries, religion and conservatism were not always linked in the same way.

At first, I was convinced that if a large portion of a country's population subscribed to an organized religion, that country would have more restrictive abortion laws mirroring trends in Christian regions of the United States. This was true in many cases. For example, Egypt, Iraq and the Philippines ban abortion under all circumstances and all three countries have a substantial majority that belongs to an Abrahamic religion (i.e. Christianity, Islam, or Judaism). However, Laos is a majority Buddhist country with a total abortion ban. In Jamaica, a relatively small 83% of the population identifies as religious, and also prohibits pregnancy termination in all cases.

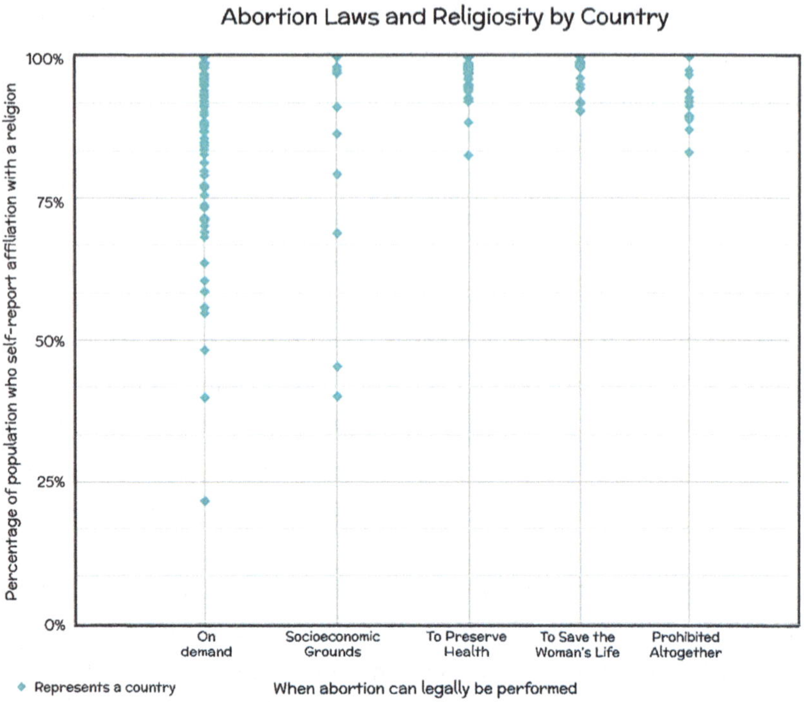

1. World Population Review. (2023). Least Religious Countries 2023. Least religious countries 2023. https://worldpopulationreview.com/country-rankings/least-religious-countries
2. The world's abortion laws. Center for Reproductive Rights. (2023, April 21). https://reproductiverights.org/-maps/worlds-abortion-laws/

The only commonality that seems to exist between religion and abortion on an international scale is that countries with less religious populations do tend to have more lenient abortion policies. However, highly religious societies aren't necessarily more likely to ban abortion, as you can see by the large number of countries that allow abortion on request and also have more than 90% of their population self-reporting as religious.

Next, I explored the idea that abortions rights are a freedom issue.[130] Surely a more "free" country would allow a broader scope for reproductive rights. After all, Egypt, Iraq and the Philippines rank as "not free" on the Freedom House Global Freedom Index Report and those countries also have full abortion bans.

When applied abroad, this theory proved only partially true. The majority of countries with full abortion bans are either categorized as "not free" or "partially free". Only 25% are ranked in the "free" category.

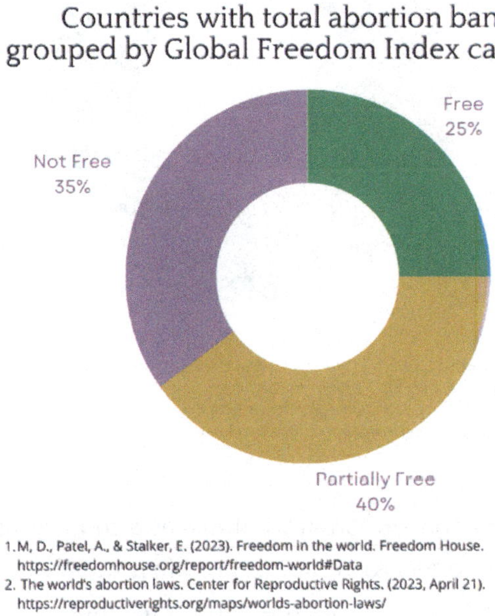

While it seems that countries with total bans are more likely to have less freedom, it does *not* appear to hold true that countries with liberal abortion laws universally have more freedom. A higher percentage of

---

[130] Schalet A. T. (2011). Beyond abstinence and risk: a new paradigm for adolescent sexual health. *Women's health issues : official publication of the Jacobs Institute of Women's Health*, *21*(3 Suppl), S5–S7. https://doi.org/10.1016/j.whi.2011.01.007https://apps.who.int/iris/bitstream/handle/10665/338768/factsheet-dpr%20korea-eng.pdf?sequence=4&isAllowed=y#:~:text=In%20October%202015%2C%20North%20Korean,the%20country's%20falling%20birth%20rate%20.&text=The%20Democratic%20People's%20Republic%20(DPR,part%20of%20the%20Korean%20Peninsula.

countries with legalized abortion-on-request are categorized as "free". However, if we combine the number of countries that fall into "not free" or "partly free" categories, it breaks down to about 50% free and about 50% not. A half/half split is not particularly noteworthy.

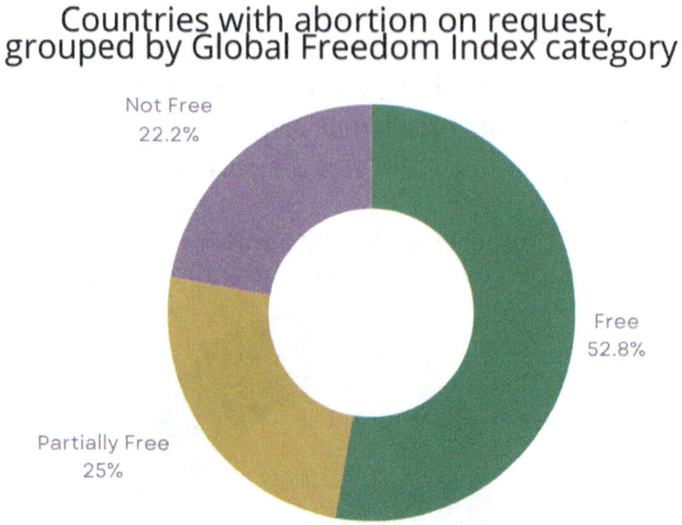

1. M, D., Patel, A., & Stalker, E. (2023). Freedom in the world. Freedom House. https://freedomhouse.org/report/freedom-world#Data
2. The world's abortion laws. Center for Reproductive Rights. (2023, April 21). https://reproductiverights.org/maps/worlds-abortion-laws/

It turns out that our conception of what makes a country, or even a person, more likely to be pro-choice or pro-life is not always applicable on a global scale. That being said, there are some international trends that seem to cross borders.

1. Abortion laws are becoming more permissive worldwide. The idea that 'abortion rights are human rights' is becoming more prevalent and we can see that being reflected in policy changes on a global scale.

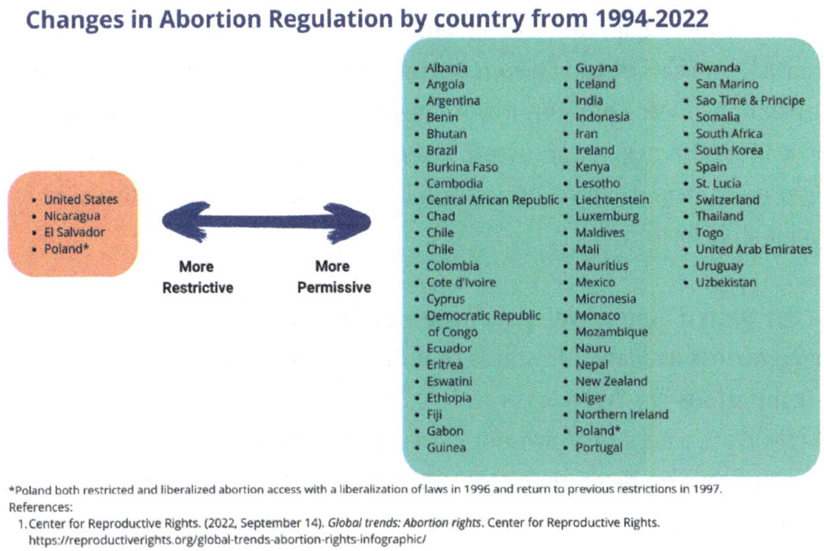

2. Self-managed medical abortion is becoming more accessible, even in countries with abortion bans. The act of outlawing abortion is now having slightly less effect than it did in the past.

For example, Nicaragua criminalizes all aspects of abortion. However, women in the region report having reliable access to abortifacient medication, misoprostol, sold under the name Cytotec and ACE Miso at most pharmacies. If you remember, misoprostol can also be used as a stomach ulcer medication, making it commonly available under that use-case. In many countries, simply claiming a history of "ulcers" may be enough to get a few pills.[131]

In a typical medication-managed abortion, both misoprostol and mifepristone are given. By using misoprostol only, one study found that 93% of pregnancies were no longer viable after medication administration. However, only 73% of pregnancies were terminated

---

[131] De Zordo, Silvia. (2016). The biomedicalisation of illegal abortion: The double life of misoprostol in Brazil. História, Ciências, Saúde-Manguinhos. 23. 19-36. 10.1590/S0104-59702016000100003.

without the need for surgical intervention (the remaining 27% needed additional medical attention to remove the remaining contents of the uterus). The same study also reported that "surgical intervention was substantially less common if women were permitted to take at least four doses [of 800 mcg misoprostol], if these doses were taken over an interval of more than 48 hours, and if the tablets were moistened before [vaginal] insertion."[132]

In the United States, we're seeing a similar situation arise as D&Cs become less available. In states that do not allow abortion procedures, organizations like Aid Access (https://aidaccess.org/en/i-need-an-abortion) will mail women abortifacient medications to take at home. With the advent of telemedicine, women can receive a consultation with instructions on how to take the pills along with follow up calls if bleeding or other side effects become a concern. Because only a few pills are needed, it's unlikely any ban on mailing medications would be effective since these pills can be easily hidden in unmarked packaging or disguised as other drugs (for example, ulcer treatments).

3. Abortion access isn't the only thing that determines abortion rates. Prenatal screening for genetic disorders coupled with decreased stigma surrounding termination leads to more terminations of pregnancies with fetal anomalies.

Abortion rights do not exist independently of other reproductive rights and regulations. Screening and genetic testing is an oft overlooked piece of the puzzle. For example, in countries with easy access to abortion and standard prenatal screening for fetal anomalies, we see the majority of pregnancies with trisomy or neural tube defects are terminated. The best examples of this effect are found in France, Belgium, Denmark,

---

[132]Raymond, E. G., Harrison, M. S., & Weaver, M. A. (2019). Efficacy of Misoprostol Alone for First-Trimester Medical Abortion: A Systematic Review. *Obstetrics and gynecology, 133*(1), 137–147. https://doi.org/10.1097/AOG.0000000000003017

Spain and Switzerland (additional countries have similar screening and abortion rates, but it was difficult to find definitive data from their governments, so only the countries with easy access to data are included in this discussion).

All of these countries offer both a nuchal translucency screening around 11-13 weeks and a maternal serum test between 8-14 weeks of pregnancy, regardless of maternal age or risk factors, both of which help screen for trisomies.[133] If significant risk factors or abnormal screening tests are present, more extensive testing like amniocentesis or chorionic villus sampling are offered which can diagnose a large swatch of genetic abnormalities and neural tube defects. Additionally, all screening is covered by government healthcare and comes at no cost to the woman.

In Denmark and Belgium, termination of pregnancy for fetal anomaly (TOPFA) is allowed up to 12 weeks with no supporting evidence from a physician, and after 12 weeks if agreed upon by two physicians. In Spain, it's legal until 22 weeks and if major defects are observed, later term terminations may be allowed. Switzerland has no legal limit on termination although almost all procedures happen before 24 weeks, and France has no restriction on ending a pregnancy with trisomy. Largely due to these guidelines, the amount of live births that occur for Trisomy 13 or 18 are well under 1 birth/100,000. If we track Trisomy 21, we can see that from 1990, the percentage of pregnancies found to have a third chromosome 21 that were aborted continues to rise. Many people now question if Down Syndrome will be eliminated in future populations.[134]

---

[133] EUROCAT. (2010). (rep.). *Prenatal Screening Policies in Europe 2010.* Retrieved July 7, 2023, from https://www.orpha.net/actor/Orphanews/2010/doc/Special-Report-Prenatal-Screening-Policies.pdf.

[134] *European platform on Rare disease registration*. European Commission. (2023, June). https://eu-rd-platform.jrc.ec.europa.eu/eurocat/eurocat-data/prevalence_en

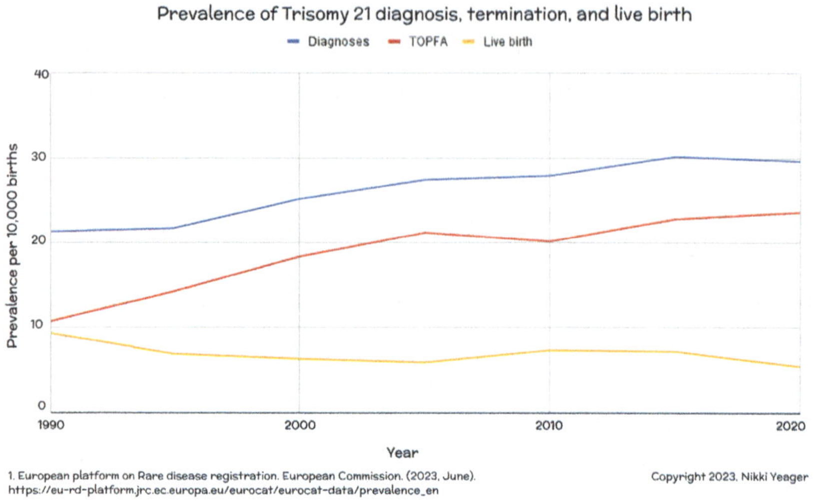

If a person chooses to have a baby with a trisomy or neural tube defect, what are the consequences? It turns out the cost of raising children with Down Syndrome may be overestimated with one study showing that the average uptick in monthly costs for a family with a child who has Trisomy 21 is only $84 a month.[135] The remainder of the cost is typically covered by insurance considering medical treatments and even things like Occupational Therapy may be covered by an insurance provider.

However, not every family has access to insurance in the United States, especially those who are self employed and/or work exclusively as freelancers/contractors. In that case, the additional cost per month over the first 18 years of life would be astronomically high considering a single visit to a pediatrician typically starts around $100 without any special therapy or treatment.

This is where we must acknowledge that the American system is unique to most developed countries in that we have privatized healthcare. Unlike countries with standardized healthcare, an American mother's

---

[135] Kageleiry A, Samuelson D, Duh MS, Lefebvre P, Campbell J, Skotko BG. 2016. Out-of-pocket medical costs and third-party healthcare costs for children with Down syndrome. Am J Med Genet Part A 9999A:1–11.

access to prenatal care and, later, assistance for a special needs child is drastically different based on her home state, income level, and employment. This is relevant when it comes to comparing reproductive health because many people without easy access to prenatal care may avoid routine visits to a gynecologist during pregnancy due to out-of-pocket expenses and lost wages. By delaying care until the second trimester, any screening that would be done for fetal abnormalities is delayed until after the point most states allow abortion in a post-Roe v. Wade world. Additionally, without regular OBGYN visits, a person may not be educated on preventive measures like taking prenatal vitamins before, and during, a pregnancy, without which the rate of neural tube defects increases. If she happens to have a baby with severe spina bifida due to a lack of prenatal folate, she may not know until the birth of the child if she did not receive routine screening. Once she gives birth, she may not have the financial ability to pay for services that keep her child healthy or the time resources to provide him/her the extra care they need. Unfortunately for her, the majority of adoptive families are not open to adopting a physically or mentally impaired infant. In this case, is early screening and abortion-on-request a better alternative?

How does the United States compare overall?

As I write this book in 2023, the state of abortion and reproductive rights is largely in flux. Additional laws are being debated regarding more restrictive abortion bans in some states, while others are moving towards a more permissive approach. There have also been rumors that topics like emergency contraceptives and birth control are going to be entering public debate again in the coming years. We'll just have to wait and see.

In the meantime, use this book to go out and argue your point. Take a stand for, or against, whatever law you'd like, but do it in a medically accurate way now that you've learned the facts.

And remember, no matter how heated, let's end our debates the same way we expect children to end intense football games – with a handshake and some common decency.

References

1. Abortion. (2022). In *Merriam-Webster.com.* Retrieved August 12, 2022, from https://www.merriam-webster.com/dictionary/abortion.
2. Abma, J. C., & Martinez, G. M. (2017). Sexual activity and contraceptive use among teenagers in the United States, 2011–2015. National health statistics reports; no 104. Hyattsville, MD: National Center for Health Statistics. 2017.
3. Adair, M. J. (1995). Plato's View of the "Wandering Uterus." *The Classical Journal, 91*(2), 153–163. http://www.jstor.org/stable/3298478
4. African Commission on Human and Peoples' Rights. (2003). (rep.). *PROTOCOL TO THE AFRICAN CHARTER ON HUMAN AND PEOPLES' RIGHTS ON THE RIGHTS OF WOMEN IN AFRICA*. Retrieved July 6, 2023, from https://www.ohchr.org/sites/default/files/Documents/Issues/Women/WG/ProtocolontheRightsofWomen.pdf.
5. Ahlgren, M. (2010). Sperm Transport to and Survival in the Human Fallopian Tube. *Gynecologic and Obstetric Investigation, 6*(3-4), 206-214.
6. Allen, R., James, A., & Sankaran, S. (2021). Trends in termination of pregnancy for neural tube defects in England and Wales from 2007 to 2017: observational prospective study. *Prenat Diagn, 41*(13), 1624-1633. https://doi.org/10.1002/pd.6060
7. American Heart Association. (2023). (rep.). *CARES Annual 2022 Report*. American Heart Association. Retrieved July 6, 2023, from https://mycares.net/sitepages/uploads/2023/2022_flipbook/index.html?page=1.

8. Aminimoghaddam, S., & Maghsoudnia, A. (2017). Unusual Presentation of Invasive Mole: A Case Report. *Journal of reproduction & infertility*, *18*(1), 205–209.
9. Amnesty International. (2021, June 23). *Egypt: Military pledges to stop forced "virginity tests."* Amnesty International. https://www.amnesty.org/en/latest/press-release/2011/06/egypt-military-pledges-stop-forced-virginity-tests/
10. Annan, J. J., Gudi, A., Bhide, P., Shah, A., & Homburg, R. (2013). Biochemical pregnancy during assisted conception: a little bit pregnant. *Journal of clinical medicine research*, *5*(4), 269–274. https://doi.org/10.4021/jocmr1008w
11. Archambault, J. (2007) .Time Limits for Conducting a Forensic Examination: Can Biological Evidence be Recovered 24, 36, 48, 72, 84 or 96 Hours Following a Sexual Assault? Sexual Assault Report, Civic Research Institute Inc., Kingston, NJ, Volume 10, Number 3, January/February 2007, p 33-47
12. Badr, S., Ghareep, A., Abdulla, L. M., & Hassanein, R. (2013). Ectopic pregnancy in uncommon implantation sites. *The Egyptian Journal of Radiology and Nuclear Medicine, 44,* 121–130. https://doi.org/10.1016/j.ejrnm.2012.10.006
13. Baicker, K., & Chandra, A. (2004). Medicare spending, the physician workforce, and beneficiaries' quality of care. *Health Aff (Millwood), 23*(suppl W4), 184-197.
14. Bayer Healthcare Pharmaceuticals. Mirena [package insert]. U.S. Food and Drug Administration website. https://www.accessdata.fda.gov/drugsatfda_docs/label/2008/021225s019lbl.pdf. Published 2018. Accessed 22/6/2023.
15. Bell, E. F., Hintz, S. R., Hansen, N. I., et al. (2022). Mortality, In-Hospital Morbidity, Care Practices, and 2-Year Outcomes for Extremely Preterm Infants in the US, 2013-2018. *JAMA, 327*(3), 248–263. doi:10.1001/jama.2021.23580
16. Berg, S. (2020, December 16). *Why stigma prevents treating menstrual hygiene as essential.* American Medical Association. https://www.ama-assn.org/delivering-care/population-care/why-stigma-prevents-treating-menstrual-hygiene-essential
17. Beriwal, S., Impey, L., & Ioannou, C. (2020). Multifetal pregnancy reduction and selective termination. *The Obstetrician & Gynaecologist, 22*, 284–292. https://doi.org/10.1111/tog.12690

18. Blencowe, H., Kancherla, V., Moorthie, S., Darlison, M.W., & Modell, B. (2018). Estimates of global and regional prevalence of neural tube defects for 2015: a systematic analysis. *Ann. N.Y. Acad. Sci., 1414,* 31-46. https://doi.org/10.1111/nyas.13548
19. Braddock, B., McDaniel, J., Spragge, S., Loncke, F., Braddock, S. R., & Carey, J. C. (2012). Communication Ability in Persons with Trisomy 18 and Trisomy 13. *Augmentative and Alternative Communication, 28*(4), 266-277. doi: 10.3109/07434618.2012.706637
20. Bureau of Justice Statistics. (2000). (rep.). *Sexual Assault of Young Children as Reported to Law Enforcement: Victim, Incident, and Offender Characteristics*. Retrieved July 6, 2023, from https://bjs.ojp.gov/library/publications/sexual-assault-young-children-reported-law-enforcement-victim-incident-and.
21. Calhaz-Jorge, C., and others. (2020). Survey on ART and IUI: legislation, regulation, funding and registries in European countries: The European IVF-monitoring Consortium (EIM) for the European Society of Human Reproduction and Embryology (ESHRE), *Human Reproduction Open, 2020*(1), hoz044, https://doi.org/10.1093/hropen/hoz044
22. Campoamor, D. (2021, June 25). *Marjorie Taylor Greene is as wrong about plan B as she is about everything else*. Does Marjorie Taylor Greene Know What Plan B Is? https://www.refinery29.com/en-us/2021/06/10546850/marjorie-taylor-greene-plan-b-abortion-pill-difference
23. Campoamor, D. (2021, June 25). *Marjorie Taylor Greene is as wrong about plan B as she is about everything else*. Does Marjorie Taylor Greene Know What Plan B Is? https://www.refinery29.com/en-us/2021/06/10546850/marjorie-taylor-greene-plan-b-abortion-pill-difference
24. Caputo, L., Cornara, L., Raimondo, F. M., De Feo, V., Vanin, S., Denaro, M., Trombetta, D., & Smeriglio, A. (2021). *Mentha pulegium* L.: A Plant Underestimated for Its Toxicity to Be Recovered from the Perspective of the Circular Economy. *Molecules (Basel, Switzerland), 26*(8), 2154. https://doi.org/10.3390/molecules26082154
25. CAT Committee, *Concluding Observations: Nicaragua*, para. 16, U.N. Doc. CAT/C/NIC/CO/1 (2009); CAT Committee, *Concluding Observations: Peru*, para. 23, U.N. Doc. CAT/C/PER/CO/4 (2006).

26. CBS. (2015, February 24). *Idaho lawmaker asks if swallowing small camera could allow remote gynecological exams*. CBS News. https://www.cbsnews.com/sanfrancisco/news/idaho-lawmaker-asks-if-swallowing-small-camera-could-allow-remote-gynecological-exams/
27. Center for Biologics Evaluation and Research. (2018, February 2). *Anthrax*. U.S. Food and Drug Administration. https://www.fda.gov/vaccines-blood-biologics/vaccines/anthrax#:~:text=The%20mortality%20rates%20from%20anthrax,that%20is%2080%25%20or%20higher.
28. Centers for Disease Control and Prevention. (2023, April 11). *STD facts - congenital syphilis*. Centers for Disease Control and Prevention. https://www.cdc.gov/std/syphilis/stdfact-congenital-syphilis.htm#:~:text=What%20is%20congenital%20syphilis%20(CS,Learn%20more%20about%20syphilis.
29. Centers for Disease Control and Prevention. 2020 Assisted Reproductive Technology Fertility Clinic and National Summary Report. US Dept of Health and Human Services; 2022.
30. Centers for Disease Control and Prevention. (2023, May 15). *Facts about hypertension*. Centers for Disease Control and Prevention. https://www.cdc.gov/bloodpressure/facts.htm#:~:text=Nearly%20half%20of%20adults%20in,are%20taking%20medication%20for%20hypertension.
31. Chattopadhyay, P., Magdanz, V., Hernández-Meliá, M., Borchert, K. B. L., Schwarz, D., & Simmchen, J. (2022), Size-Dependent Inhibition of Sperm Motility by Copper Particles as a Path toward Male Contraception. *Adv. NanoBiomed Res., 2*, 2100152. https://doi.org/10.1002/anbr.202100152
32. Chaudhry, K., Tafti, D., Siccardi, M. A. Anembryonic Pregnancy. [Updated 2023 May 22]. In: StatPearls [Internet]. Treasure Island (FL): StatPearls Publishing; 2023 Jan-. Available from: https://www.ncbi.nlm.nih.gov/books/NBK499938/
33. Cheng, T. L., Mistry, K. B., Wang, G., Zuckerman, B., & Wang, X. (2018). Folate Nutrition Status in Mothers of the Boston Birth Cohort, Sample of a US Urban Low-Income Population. *American journal of public health, 108*(6), 799–807. https://doi.org/10.2105/AJPH.2018.304355

34. Clearblue. (2023, May 2). *When can I take a pregnancy test?* Clearblue. https://www.clearblue.com/pregnancy-tests/early-pregnancy-testing
35. CNY Fertility. (2021, December 2). *Donor Egg Cost & financing: The average cost of donor egg IVF in USA*. CNY Fertility. https://www.cnyfertility.com/donor-egg-cost/#costs-of-infertility-treatment-results-from-an-18-month-prospective-cohort-study
36. Cook, T., Bruner, B., Trombly, M., & Eom, D. (2022, July 26). *Ohio man charged in rape of 10-year-old that led to Indiana abortion*. The Indianapolis Star. https://www.indystar.com/story/news/2022/07/13/ohio-man-charged-rape-10-year-old-led-indiana-abortion/10048529002/
37. Cooper, D. B., Patel, P., & Mahdy, H. (2023). Oral Contraceptive Pills. [Updated 2022 Nov 24]. In: StatPearls [Internet]. Treasure Island (FL): StatPearls Publishing; 2023 Jan-. Available from: https://www.ncbi.nlm.nih.gov/books/NBK430882/
38. Copeland, L. (2017, June 15). *From medical pariah to feminist icon: The story of the IUD*. Smithsonian.com. https://www.smithsonianmag.com/science-nature/medical-pariah-feminist-icon-story-iud-180963699/
39. Cui, J., Shen, Y., & Li, R. (2013). Estrogen synthesis and signaling pathways during aging: from periphery to brain. *Trends in molecular medicine, 19*(3), 197–209. https://doi.org/10.1016/j.molmed.2012.12.007
40. Dacaj, R., Izetbegovic, S., Stojkanovic, G., & Dreshaj, S. (2016). Elevated Liver Enzymes in Cases of Preeclampsia and Intrauterine Growth Restriction. *Medical archives (Sarajevo, Bosnia and Herzegovina), 70*(1), 44–47. https://doi.org/10.5455/medarh.2016.70.44-47
41. De Zordo, Silvia. (2016). The biomedicalisation of illegal abortion: The double life of misoprostol in Brazil. *História, Ciências, Saúde-Manguinhos*. 23. 19-36. 10.1590/S0104-59702016000100003.
42. Debnath, J., Gulati, S. K., Mathur, A., Gupta, R., Kumar, N., Arora, S., & Krishna, R. B. (2013). Ectopic pregnancy in the era of medical abortion: are we ready for it? Spectrum of sonographic findings and our experience in a tertiary care service hospital of

India. *J Obstet Gynaecol India, 63*(6), 388-393. doi: 10.1007/s13224-013-0459-2
43. Donovan, K. A., An, J., Nowak, R. P., Yuan, J. C., Fink, E. C., Berry, B. C., Ebert, B. L., & Fischer, E. S. (2018) Thalidomide promotes degradation of SALL4, a transcription factor implicated in Duane Radial Ray syndrome eLife 7:e38430. https://doi.org/10.7554/eLife.38430
44. Driscoll, D. (2004). The Professional Practice and Guidelines Committee. Second trimester maternal serum screening for fetal open neural tube defects and aneuploidy. *Genet Med, 6*, 540–541. https://doi.org/10.1097/00125817-200411000-00013
45. Duncan, F. E., Schindler, K., Schultz, R. M., Blengini, C. S., Stein, P., Stricker, S. A., Wessel, G. M., & Williams, C. J. (2020). Unscrambling the oocyte and the egg: clarifying terminology of the female gamete in mammals. *Molecular human reproduction, 26*(11), 797–800. https://doi.org/10.1093/molehr/gaaa066
46. Edwards, M., & Can, A. S. (2023). Progestin. [Updated 2023 Mar 11]. In: StatPearls [Internet]. Treasure Island (FL): StatPearls Publishing; 2023 Jan-. Available from: https://www.ncbi.nlm.nih.gov/books/NBK563211/
47. Emergency contraception. (2015). Practice Bulletin No. 152. American College of Obstetricians and Gynecologists. *Obstet Gynecol, 126*, e1–11.
48. Etienne, V. (2023, February 27). *Jessa Duggar says she had a D&C, how does that differ from other abortion procedures?* Peoplemag. https://people.com/health/jessa-duggar-d-and-c-differ-from-other-abortions/
49. European League Against Rheumatism. (2015, June 11). Non-steroidal anti-inflammatory drugs inhibit ovulation after just 10 days. *ScienceDaily*. Retrieved June 21, 2023 from www.sciencedaily.com/releases/2015/06/150611082124.htm
50. European Medicines Agency. (2009). (rep.). *CHMP ASSESSMENT REPORT FOR EllaOne*. Retrieved July 6, 2023, from https://www.ema.europa.eu/en/documents/assessment-report/ellaone-epar-public-assessment-report_en.pdf.
51. *European platform on Rare disease registration*. European Commission. (2023, June). https://eu-rd-platform.jrc.ec.europa.eu/eurocat/eurocat-data/prevalence_en

52. *Evaluating ulipristal acetate and misoprostol for induced abortion through 63 days of pregnancy*. ISRCTNregistry. (2022, September 2). https://www.isrctn.com/ISRCTN35625202
53. Ferré-sadurní, L. (2019, December 3). *After the rapper T.I.'s remarks, N.Y. may ban "virginity tests."* The New York Times. https://www.nytimes.com/2019/12/03/nyregion/virginity-test-ti-ny-law.html
54. Frank, J. (2016, June 10). *Bob Beauprez's IUD Remark in debate generates controversy*. The Denver Post. https://www.denverpost.com/2014/10/01/bob-beauprezs-iud-remark-in-debate-generates-controversy/
55. Gallion, H. R., Milam, L. J., & Littrell, L. L. (2016). Genital Findings in Cases of Child Sexual Abuse: Genital vs Vaginal Penetration. *Journal of pediatric and adolescent gynecology*, *29*(6), 604–611. https://doi.org/10.1016/j.jpag.2016.05.001
56. Gemzell-Danielsson, K., Mansour, D., Fiala, C., Kaunitz, A. M., & Bahamondes, L. (2013). Management of pain associated with the insertion of intrauterine contraceptives. *Human reproduction update*, *19*(4), 419–427. https://doi.org/10.1093/humupd/dmt022
57. Grady, W. R., & Tanfer, K. (1994). Condom breakage and slippage among men in the United States. *Family planning perspectives*, *26*(3), 107–112.
58. Grenoble, R. (2022, August 11). *Meet the Utah councilor who thinks "a baby is not part of the body of a woman."* HuffPost. https://www.huffpost.com/entry/david-alvord-utah-abortion-reproductive-rights_n_62f51c13e4b0da517ef67194
59. Hajji, A., Toumi, D., Laakom, O., Cherif, O., & Faleh, R. (2020). Early primary abdominal pregnancy: Diagnosis and management. A case report. *International journal of surgery case reports*, *73*, 303–306. https://doi.org/10.1016/j.ijscr.2020.07.048
60. Han, L., Padua, E., Hart, K. D., Edelman, A., & Jensen, J. T. (2019). Comparing cervical mucus changes in response to an oral progestin or oestrogen withdrawal in ovarian-suppressed women: a clinical pilot. *The European journal of contraception & reproductive health care: the official journal of the European Society of Contraception*, *24*(3), 209–215. https://doi.org/10.1080/13625187.2019.1605503

61. Hannon, P. (2022, May 19). *Stanford biomedical ethicists among panelists updating law on definition of death*. Stanford Medicine News Center. https://med.stanford.edu/news/all-news/2022/05/definition-death-law.html
62. Holesh, J. E., Bass, A. N., & Lord, M. (2023). Physiology, Ovulation. [Updated 2023 May 1]. In: StatPearls [Internet]. Treasure Island (FL): StatPearls Publishing; 2023 Jan-. Available from: https://www.ncbi.nlm.nih.gov/books/NBK441996/
63. Hopkins, C. (2022, June 25). *The 'abortion pill' may treat a disease affecting many veterans. what happens now?* NBCNews.com. Retrieved August 1, 2022, from https://www.nbcnews.com/health/health-news/abortion-pill-may-treat-dozens-diseases-roe-reversal-might-upend-resea-rcna34812
64. Human Fertilisation and Embryology Authority. (n.d.). *Approved PGT-M and PTT conditions*. HFEA. https://www.hfea.gov.uk/treatments/embryo-testing-and-treatments-for-disease/approved-pgt-m-and-ptt-conditions/
65. Human Rights Committee, *General Comment No. 36 (2018) on Article 6 of the International Covenant on Civil and Political Rights, on the Right to Life*, at 2, para. 8, U.N. Doc. CCPR/C/GC/36 (2018)
66. Institute of Medicine (US) Committee to Study Decision Making; Hanna KE, editor. Biomedical Politics. Washington (DC): National Academies Press (US); 1991. A Political History of RU-486. Available from: https://www.ncbi.nlm.nih.gov/books/NBK234199/
67. Jenny, C., Kuhns, M. L., & Arakawa, F. (1987). Hymens in newborn female infants. *Pediatrics, 80*(3), 399-400. PMID: 3627892.
68. Jesam, C., Salvatierra, A. M., Schwartz, J. L., Fuentes, A., & Croxatto, H. B. (2014). Effect of oral administration of a continuous 18 day regimen of meloxicam on ovulation: experience of a randomized controlled trial. *Contraception, 90*(2), 168–173. https://doi.org/10.1016/j.contraception.2014.04.011
69. Joensuu-Manninen, H., Kuvaja, P. & Talvensaari-Mattila, A. (2010), Clinical efficacy of mifepristone and misoprostol in second trimester pregnancy termination. *Acta Obstetricia et*

Gynecologica Scandinavica, 89, 1552-1556. https://doi.org/10.3109/00016349.2010.513427

70. Jones, R. K., Guttmacher Institute, Nash, E., Cross, L., Philbin, J., & Kirstein, M. (2022, July 14). *Medication abortion now accounts for more than half of all US abortions*. Guttmacher Institute. Retrieved August 1, 2022, from https://www.guttmacher.org/article/2022/02/medication-abortion-now-accounts-more-half-all-us-abortions
71. Jones, J. S., Wynn, B. N., Kroeze, B., Dunnuck, C., & Rossman, L. (2004). Comparison of sexual assaults by strangers versus known assailants in a community-based population. *The American journal of emergency medicine, 22*(6), 454–459. https://doi.org/10.1016/j.ajem.2004.07.020
72. Kadanali, S., Küçüközkan, T., Zor, N., Kumtepe, Y. (1996). Comparison of labor induction with misoprostol vs. oxytocin/prostaglandin E2 in term pregnancy. *Int J Gynaecol Obstet, 55*(2), 99-104. doi: 10.1016/s0020-7292(96)02710-5
73. Kageleiry, A., Samuelson, D., Duh, M. S., Lefebvre, P., Campbell J, & Skotko, B. G. (2016). Out-of-pocket medical costs and third-party healthcare costs for children with Down syndrome. *Am J Med Genet. Part A, 9999A*, 1–11.
74. Kakinuma, T., Kakinuma, K., Sakamoto, Y., Kawarai, Y., Saito, K., Ihara, M., Matsuda, Y., Sato, I., Ohwada, M., Yanagida, K., & Tanaka, H. (2020). Safety and efficacy of manual vacuum suction compared with conventional dilatation and sharp curettage and electric vacuum aspiration in surgical treatment of miscarriage: a randomized controlled trial. *BMC Pregnancy Childbirth, 20*(1), 695. doi: 10.1186/s12884-020-03362-4
75. Katz, A. (2018, July 19). *Sex ed goes global: The Netherlands*. Global Reproductive Health at Duke. https://dukecenterforglobalreproductivehealth.org/2018/07/19/sex-ed-goes-global-the-netherlands/
76. Kortsmit, K., Nguyen, A. T., Mandel, M. G., et al. (2022). Abortion Surveillance — United States, 2020. *MMWR Surveill Summ, 71*(No. SS-10):1–27. http://dx.doi.org/10.15585/mmwr.ss7110a1
77. Lira-Albarrán, S., Durand, M., Barrera, D., Vega, C., Becerra, R. G., Díaz, L., García-Quiroz, J., Rangel, C., & Larrea, F. (2018). A single preovulatory administration of ulipristal acetate affects the decidualization process of the human endometrium during

the receptive period of the menstrual cycle. *Molecular and cellular endocrinology*, *476*, 70–78. https://doi.org/10.1016/j.mce.2018.04.010

78. Lorthe, E., Torchin, H., Delorme, P., Ancel, P. Y., Marchand-Martin, L., Foix-L'Hélias, L., Benhammou, V., Gire, C., d'Ercole, C., Winer, N., Sentilhes, L., Subtil, D., Goffinet, F., & Kayem, G. (2018). Preterm premature rupture of membranes at 22-25 weeks' gestation: perinatal and 2-year outcomes within a national population-based study (EPIPAGE-2). *American journal of obstetrics and gynecology*, *219*(3), 298.e1–298.e14. https://doi.org/10.1016/j.ajog.2018.05.029
79. Lurie, S. (1992). The history of the diagnosis and treatment of ectopic pregnancy: a medical adventure. *European journal of obstetrics, gynecology, and reproductive biology*, *43*(1), 1–7. https://doi.org/10.1016/0028-2243(92)90235-q
80. Marchione, M. (2019, January 17). *In limbo: Leftover embryos challenge clinics, couples*. AP NEWS. https://apnews.com/article/health-north-america-us-news-ap-top-news-ca-state-wire-046d6fbc4c564caebac7e560cd87a26a
81. Martinez, G. M. (2020). Trends and patterns in menarche in the United States, 1995 through 2013–2017. National Health Statistics Reports; no 146. Hyattsville, MD: National Center for Health Statistics. 2020
82. Martinez, G., Abma, J., & Copen, C. (2010). Educating teenagers about sex in the United States. NCHS data brief, no 44. Hyattsville, MD: National Center for Health Statistics. 2010.
83. Meyer, R. E., Liu, G., Gilboa, S. M., Ethen, M. K., Aylsworth, A. S., Powell, C. M., Flood, T. J., Mai, C. T., Wang, Y., Canfield, M. A., & National Birth Defects Prevention Network. (2016). Survival of children with trisomy 13 and trisomy 18: A multi-state population-based study. *American journal of medical genetics. Part A*, *170A*(4), 825–837. https://doi.org/10.1002/ajmg.a.37495
84. Moaddab, A., McCullough, L. B., Chervenak, F. A., Stark, L., Schulkin, J., Dildy, G. A., Raine, S. P., & Shamshirsaz, A. A. (2017). A survey of honor-related practices among US obstetricians and gynecologists. *International journal of gynaecology and obstetrics: the official organ of the International Federation of Gynaecology and Obstetrics*, *139*(2), 164–169. https://doi.org/10.1002/ijgo.12294

85. Morris, J. K., & Savva, G. M. (2008). The risk of fetal loss following a prenatal diagnosis of trisomy 13 or trisomy 18. *American journal of medical genetics. Part A, 146A*(7), 827–832. https://doi.org/10.1002/ajmg.a.32220
86. Mozzanega, B., & Nardelli, G. B. (2019). UPA and LNG in emergency contraception: the information by EMA and the scientific evidences indicate a prevalent anti-implantation effect. *The European journal of contraception & reproductive health care: the official journal of the European Society of Contraception, 24*(1), 4–10. https://doi.org/10.1080/13625187.2018.1555662
87. Nada, Z. M., Assaf, N. F., Dubey, S. K., & JMC Board (2005). Human sperm can fertilize ova inside the Graafian follicles before ovulation. *Fertility and sterility, 83*(2), 457–461. https://doi.org/10.1016/j.fertnstert.2004.09.013
88. Noé, G., Croxatto, H. B., Salvatierra, A. M., Reyes, V., Villarroel, C., Muñoz, C., Morales, G., & Retamales, A. (2011). Contraceptive efficacy of emergency contraception with levonorgestrel given before or after ovulation. *Contraception, 84*(5), 486–492. https://doi.org/10.1016/j.contraception.2011.03.006
89. Novikova, N., Weisberg, E., Stanczyk, F. Z., Croxatto, H. B., & Fraser, I. S. (2007). Effectiveness of levonorgestrel emergency contraception given before or after ovulation--a pilot study. *Contraception, 75*(2), 112–118. https://doi.org/10.1016/j.contraception.2006.08.015
90. NYC Health. (2019). *What Group Child Care Providers Should Know*. NYC, NY; NYC Health. Retrieved June 23, 2023.
91. Ortiz, M. E., Croxatto, H. B., & Bardin, C. W. (1996). Mechanisms of action of intrauterine devices. *Obstetrical & gynecological survey, 51*(12 Suppl), S42–S51. https://doi.org/10.1097/00006254-199612000-00014
92. Paybarah, A. (2022, June 28). *G.O.P. house candidate falsely suggests pregnancy from rape is unlikely.* The New York Times. https://www.nytimes.com/2022/06/27/us/politics/yesli-vega-rape-pregnant.html
93. Planned Parenthood. (n.d.). *Title X: Affordable birth control and reproductive health care.* Planned Parenthood Action Fund. https://www.plannedparenthoodaction.org/issues/health-care-

equity/title-x#:~:text=Federal%20Title%20X%20funding%20was,basic%2C%20preventive%20reproductive%20health%20care.
94. Ponzo, S., Wickham, A., Bamford, R., Radovic, T., Zhaunova, L., Peven, K., Klepchukova, A., & Payne, J. L. (2022). Menstrual cycle-associated symptoms and workplace productivity in US employees: A cross-sectional survey of users of the Flo mobile phone app. *Digital health, 8,* 20552076221145852. https://doi.org/10.1177/20552076221145852
95. Popescu, A. (2018, December 15). *The octomom has proved us all wrong*. The New York Times. https://www.nytimes.com/2018/12/15/style/octomom-kids-2018.html
96. Practice Committee of the American Society for Reproductive Medicine and the Practice Committee for the Society for Assisted Reproductive Technologies. Electronic address: ASRM@asrm.org (2021). Guidance on the limits to the number of embryos to transfer: a committee opinion. *Fertility and sterility, 116*(3), 651–654. https://doi.org/10.1016/j.fertnstert.2021.06.050
97. RAINN. (n.d.). *What is a sexual assault forensic exam?* RAINN. https://www.rainn.org/articles/rape-kit
98. Raymond, E. G., Harrison, M. S., & Weaver, M. A. (2019). Efficacy of Misoprostol Alone for First-Trimester Medical Abortion: A Systematic Review. *Obstetrics and gynecology, 133*(1), 137–147. https://doi.org/10.1097/AOG.0000000000003017
99. Rodriguez, L. (2021, October 1). *20 places around the world where governments provide free period products*. Global Citizen. https://www.globalcitizen.org/en/content/free-period-products-countries-cities-worldwide/
100. Ropper, A., & Burrell, B. D. (2015). *Reaching down the Rabbit Hole: A renowned neurologist explains the mystery and drama of ... brain disease*. Griffin.
101. Roy, A. M., Konda, M., Goel, A., & Sasapu, A. (2019). Epidemiology and Factors Affecting Mortality of Hospitalized Patients with Disseminated Intravascular Coagulation in the United States. *Blood, 134* (Supplement_1), 2404. https://doi.org/10.1182/blood-2019-132071
102. S.3 - 108th Congress (2003-2004): Partial-Birth Abortion Ban Act of 2003. (2003, November 5). https://www.congress.gov/bill/108th-congress/senate-bill/3

103. Schalet, A. T. (2011). Beyond abstinence and risk: a new paradigm for adolescent sexual health. *Women's health issues: official publication of the Jacobs Institute of Women's Health, 21*(3 Suppl), S5–S7. https://doi.org/10.1016/j.whi.2011.01
104. Scutiero, G., Di Gioia, P., Spada, A., & Greco, P. (2012). Primary ovarian pregnancy and its management. *JSLS : Journal of the Society of Laparoendoscopic Surgeons, 16*(3), 492–494. https://doi.org/10.4293/108680812X13462882736385
105. Second-trimester abortion. Practice Bulletin No. 135. American College of Obstetricians and Gynecologists. *Obstet Gynecol, 121,* 1394–1406.
106. Senat, M. V., Fischer, C., & Ville, Y. (2002). Funipuncture for fetocide in late termination of pregnancy. *Prenatal diagnosis, 22*(5), 354–356. https://doi.org/10.1002/pd.290.
107. Silber, S. J. (2022, January 7). *Beating your biological clock - understanding female eggs*. The Infertility Center of St. Louis. https://www.infertile.com/infertility-101/female-infertility/beating-biological/
108. Simmons-Duffin, S. (2023, April 25). *In Oklahoma, a woman was told to wait until she's "crashing" for abortion care*. NPR. https://www.npr.org/sections/health-shots/2023/04/25/1171851775/oklahoma-woman-abortion-ban-study-shows-confusion-at-hospitals
109. Simopoulou, M., Sfakianoudis, K., Giannelou, P., Rapani, A., Maziotis, E., Tsioulou, P., Grigoriadis, S., Simopoulos, E., Mantas, D., Lambropoulou, M., Koutsilieris, M., Pantos, K., & Harper, J. C. (2019). Discarding IVF embryos: reporting on global practices. *Journal of assisted reproduction and genetics, 36*(12), 2447–2457. https://doi.org/10.1007/s10815-019-01592-w
110. Smoley, B. A., & Robinson, C. M. (2012). Natural family planning. *American family physician, 86*(10), 924–928.
111. Springer, S., Karner, E., Worda, C., Grabner, M. M., Seidl-Mlczoch, E., Laccone, F., Neesen, J., Scharrer, A., & Ulm, B. (2022). Outcome after Prenatal Diagnosis of Trisomy 13, 18, and 21 in Fetuses with Congenital Heart Disease. *Life (Basel, Switzerland), 12*(8), 1223. https://doi.org/10.3390/life12081223
112. Süzen Çaypınar, S., Oğlak, S. C., Polat, İ. *et al.* (2023*)* A new and more effective feticide technique in late termination of pregnancy: potassium chloride injection into the interventricular

septum of the fetal heart. *Arch Gynecol Obstet, 307*, 779–787. https://doi.org/10.1007/s00404-022-06795-8
113. *Teen birth rate comparison, 2020*. Teen Birth Rate Comparison, 2020 | Power to Decide. (n.d.). https://powertodecide.org/what-we-do/information/national-state-data/teen-birth-rate
114. Thomas, C., Cavazza, T., & Schuh, M. (2021). Aneuploidy in human eggs: contributions of the meiotic spindle. *Biochemical Society transactions*, *49*(1), 107–118. https://doi.org/10.1042/BST20200043
115. Tirgar, P., Sarmadi, F., Najafi, M., Kazemi, P., AzizMohseni, S., Fayazi, S., Zandi, G., Ziaie, N., Naseri, A. S. Z., Ehrlicher, A., & Dashtizad, M. (2021). Toward embryo cryopreservation-on-a-chip: A standalone microfluidic platform for gradual loading of cryoprotectants to minimize cryoinjuries. *Biomicrofluidics*; *15*(3), 034104. https://doi.org/10.1063/5.0047185
116. Travis, A. (2011, May 8). *Virginity tests for immigrants "reflected dark age prejudices" of 1970s Britain*. The Guardian. https://www.theguardian.com/uk/2011/may/08/virginity-tests-immigrants-prejudices-britain
117. Trujillo, A. Card. L. (1997, February 12). *VADEMECUM FOR CONFESSORS CONCERNING SOME ASPECTS OF THE MORALITY OF CONJUGAL LIFE*. Vademecum for confessors concerning some aspects of the morality of the conjugal life. https://www.vatican.va/roman_curia/pontifical_councils/family/documents/rc_pc_family_doc_12021997_vademecum_en.html
118. *Understanding changes in life expectancy*. Cystic Fibrosis Foundation. (n.d.). https://www.cff.org/managing-cf/understanding-changes-life-expectancy
119. *Updated Guidelines for Antiretroviral Postexposure Prophylaxis after Sexual, Injection-Drug Use, or Other Nonoccupational Exposure to HIV – United States, 2016.* MMWR Morb Mortal Wkly Rep, 2016. 65(17): p. 458.
120. U.S. Department of Health and Human Services. (2020, June 3). *Office of dietary supplements - black cohosh*. NIH Office of Dietary Supplements. https://ods.od.nih.gov/factsheets/BlackCohosh-HealthProfessional/

121. U.S. Department of Health and Human Services. (n.d.). *Pregnancy test - a thin blue line the history of the pregnancy test - office of NIH history and Stetten Museum.* National Institutes of Health. https://history.nih.gov/display/history/Pregnancy+Test+-+A+Thin+Blue+Line+The+History+of+the+Pregnancy+Test
122. *Use of Ulipristal Acetate in Induction of Second Trimester Missed Abortion*. ClinicalTrials.gov. (2021, August 4). https://clinicaltrials.gov/study/NCT04989400
123. *Virtual Mentor.* 2008;10(5):304-306. doi: 10.1001/virtualmentor.2008.10.5.cprl1-0805.
124. Wall Street Journal. (2022, July 13). *Opinion | an abortion story too good to confirm*. The Wall Street Journal. https://www.wsj.com/articles/an-abortion-story-too-good-to-confirm-joe-biden-ten-year-old-girl-indiana-ohio-caitlin-bernard-11657648618?redirect=amp
125. Wexler, P. (Ed.). (2014). *Encyclopedia of Toxicology. ScienceDirect* (3rd ed.). Elsevier Academic Press.
126. Williams, T., Mortada, R., & Porter, S. (2016). Diagnosis and Treatment of Polycystic Ovary Syndrome. *American family physician*, *94*(2), 106–113.
127. Won, R. H., Currier, R. J., Lorey, F., & Towner, D. R. (2005). The timing of demise in fetuses with trisomy 21 and trisomy 18. *Prenatal diagnosis*, *25*(7), 608–611. https://doi.org/10.1002/pd.1243

Made in the USA
Monee, IL
03 November 2026

67386698R00108